The Complete Guide to Mediterranean Seafood Recipes

Health and Tasty Seafood Recipes to Enjoy Your Diet and Boost Your Metabolism

Raymond Morton

Table of contents

Basil Garlic Salmon...................................6

Yogurt Cod Mix...................................8

Halibut and Tomatoes Mix...................................10

Parsley Salmon Mix...................................12

Cod and Veggies...................................14

Cilantro Sea Bass...................................16

Balsamic Salmon and Beans...................................18

Parsley Shrimp Mix...................................20

Chives Salmon and Olives...................................22

Lemon Salmon and Endives...................................24

Coconut Cod and Asparagus...................................26

Cumin Shrimp...................................27

Sea Bass Mix...................................29

Oregano Shrimp...................................31

Shrimp and Shallots...................................33

Shrimp and Capers Salad...................................35

Cheesy Cod Mix...................................36

Lemony Tilapia Mix...................................38

Trout and Avocado Salad...................................40

Garlic Trout...................................42

Parsley Salmon...................................44

Trout and Arugula Salad...................................46

Saffron Paprika Salmon...................................48

Shrimp and Basil Salad...................................50

Shrimp and Quinoa Salad...................................52

Crab and Cherry Tomato Salad................................54

Scallops and Scallions................................56

Dill Flounder Mix................................58

Salmon and Mango................................60

Shrimp and Radish Mix................................62

Cheesy Salmon Spread................................64

Shrimp with Artichokes and Tomatoes................66

Shrimp and Sauce................................69

Oregano Tuna and Orange................................71

Fish Curry................................73

Salmon and Carrots Mix................................75

Thyme Shrimp................................77

Chili Cumin Cod................................80

Balsamic Scallops................................83

Creamy Lime Sea Bass Mix................................85

Fish and Mushrooms Mix................................87

Salmon and Tomato Soup................................89

Cinnamon Shrimp................................91

Shrimp and Blueberries Mix................................93

Baked Trout................................95

Paprika Scallops................................97

Fish Meatballs................................99

Salmon and Eggplant Pan................................101

Mustard and Turmeric Cod................................103

Shrimp and Walnuts................................105

Cod and Corn................................107

Shrimp and Mussels Mix................................109

4

Basil Garlic Salmon

Prep time: 5 minutes I **Cooking time:** 14 minutes I **Servings:** 4

Ingredients:

- 2 tablespoons olive oil
- 4 salmon fillets, skinless
- 2 garlic cloves, minced
- A pinch of black pepper
- 2 tablespoons balsamic vinegar
- 2 tablespoons basil, chopped

Directions:

1. Heat up a pan with the olive oil, add the fish and cook for 4 minutes on each side.
2. Add the rest of the ingredients, cook everything for 6 minutes more.
3. Divide everything between plates and serve.

Nutrition info per serving: calories 300, fat 18, fiber 0.1, carbs 0.6, protein 34.7

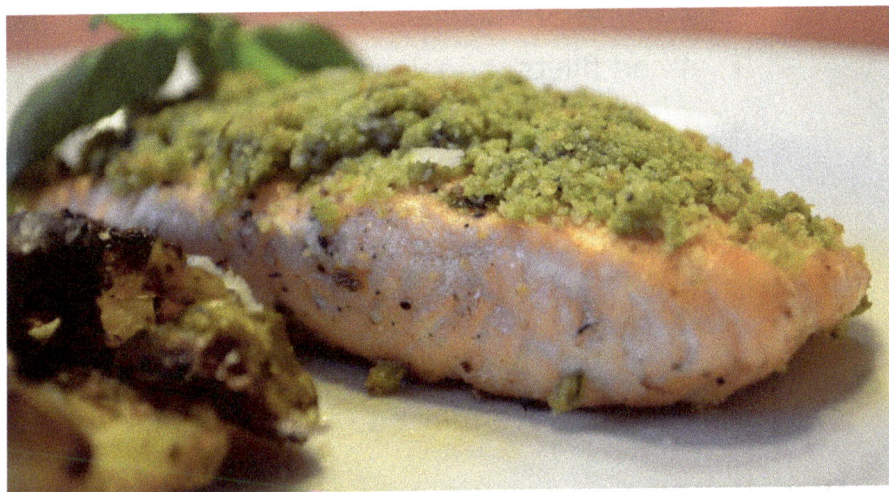

Yogurt Cod Mix

Prep time: 10 minutes I **Cooking time:** 15 minutes I
Servings: 4

Ingredients:

- 2 tablespoons olive oil
- 4 cod fillets, boneless and skinless
- 1 shallot, chopped
- ½ cup coconut cream
- 3 tablespoons Greek yogurt
- 2 tablespoons dill, chopped
- A pinch of black pepper
- 1 garlic clove minced

Directions:

1. Heat up a pan with the oil over medium heat, add the shallots and sauté for 5 minutes.
2. Add the fish and the other ingredients, and cook for 10 minutes more.
3. Divide everything between plates and serve.

Nutrition info per serving: calories 252, fat 15.2, fiber 0.9, carbs 7.7, protein 22.3

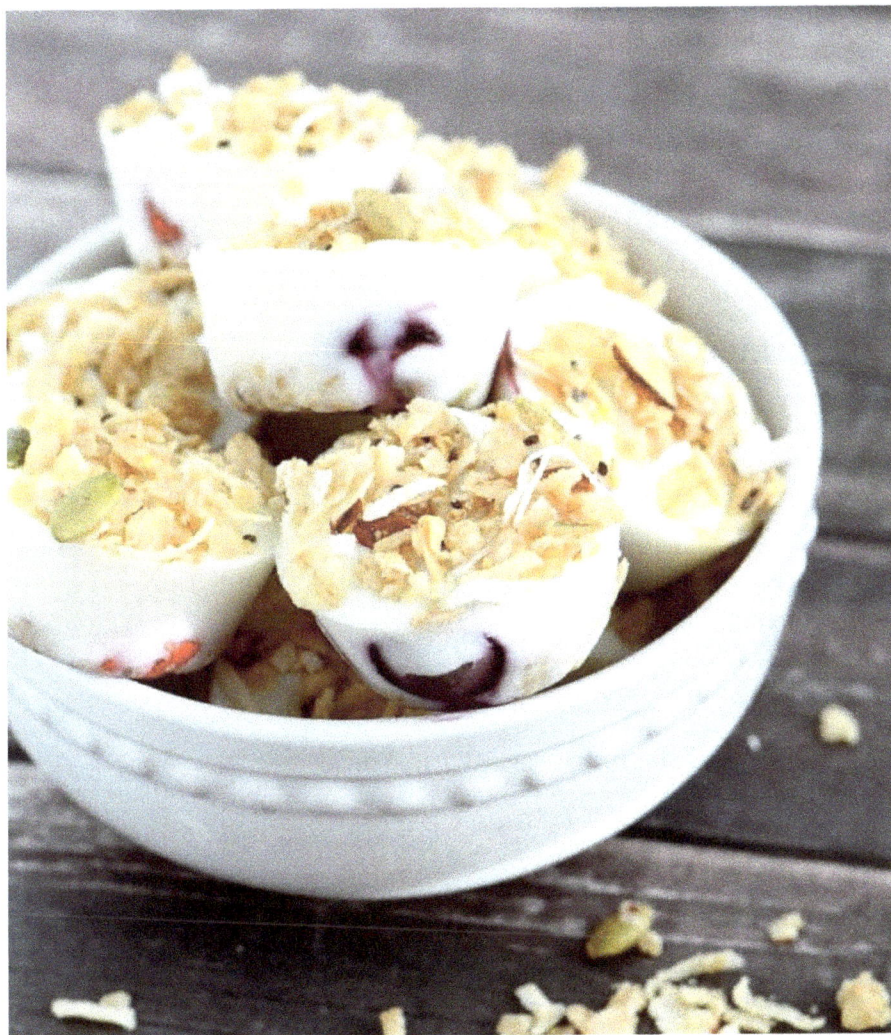

Halibut and Tomatoes Mix

Prep time: 10 minutes I **Cooking time:** 15 minutes I
Servings: 4

Ingredients:

- 2 shallots, chopped
- 4 halibut fillets, boneless
- 1 cup radishes, halved
- 1 cup tomatoes, cubed
- 1 tablespoon olive oil
- 1 tablespoon cilantro, chopped
- 2 teaspoons lemon juice
- A pinch of black pepper

Directions:

1. Grease a roasting pan with the oil and arrange the fish inside.
2. Add the rest of the ingredients, Introduce in the oven and bake at 400 degrees F for 15 minutes.
3. Divide everything between plates and serve.

Nutrition info per serving: calories 231, fat 7.8, fiber 6, carbs 11.9, protein 21.1

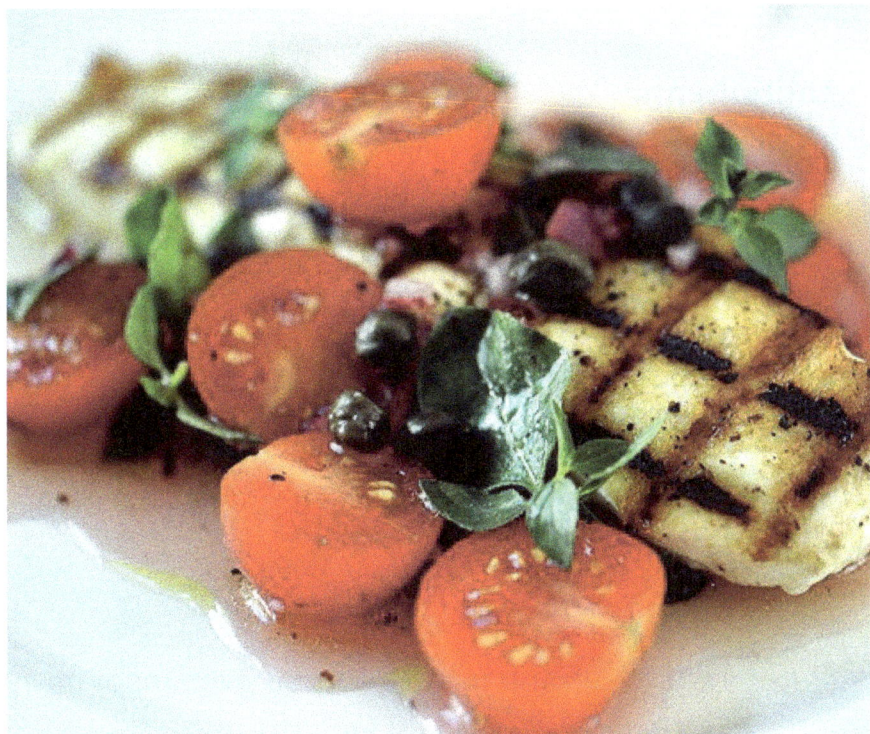

Parsley Salmon Mix

Prep time: 10 minutes I **Cooking time:** 15 minutes I
Servings: 4

Ingredients:

- 2 tablespoons olive oil
- ½ cup almonds, chopped
- 4 salmon fillets, boneless
- 1 shallot, chopped
- ½ cup veggie stock
- 2 tablespoons parsley, chopped
- Black pepper to the taste

=

Directions:

1. Heat up a pan with the oil over medium heat, add the shallot and sauté for 4 minutes.
2. Add the salmon and the other ingredients, cook for 5 minutes on each side, divide everything between plates and serve.

Nutrition info per serving: calories 240, fat 6.4, fiber 2.6, carbs 11.4, protein 15

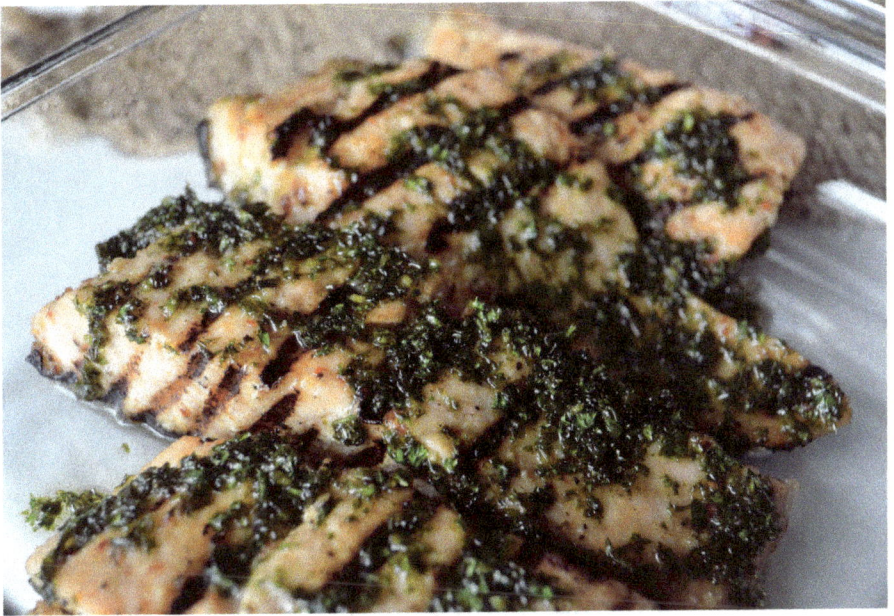

Cod and Veggies

Prep time: 10 minutes I **Cooking time:** 20 minutes I
Servings: 4

Ingredients:

- 2 tablespoons coconut aminos
- 1 pound broccoli florets
- 4 cod fillets, boneless
- 1 red onion, chopped
- 2 tablespoons olive oil
- ¼ cup chicken stock
- Black pepper to the taste

Directions:

1. Heat up a pan with the oil over medium heat, add the onion and the broccoli and cook for 5 minutes.
2. Add the fish and the other ingredients, cook for 20 minutes more, divide everything between plates and serve.

Nutrition info per serving: calories 220, fat 14.3, fiber 6.3, carbs 16.2, protein 9

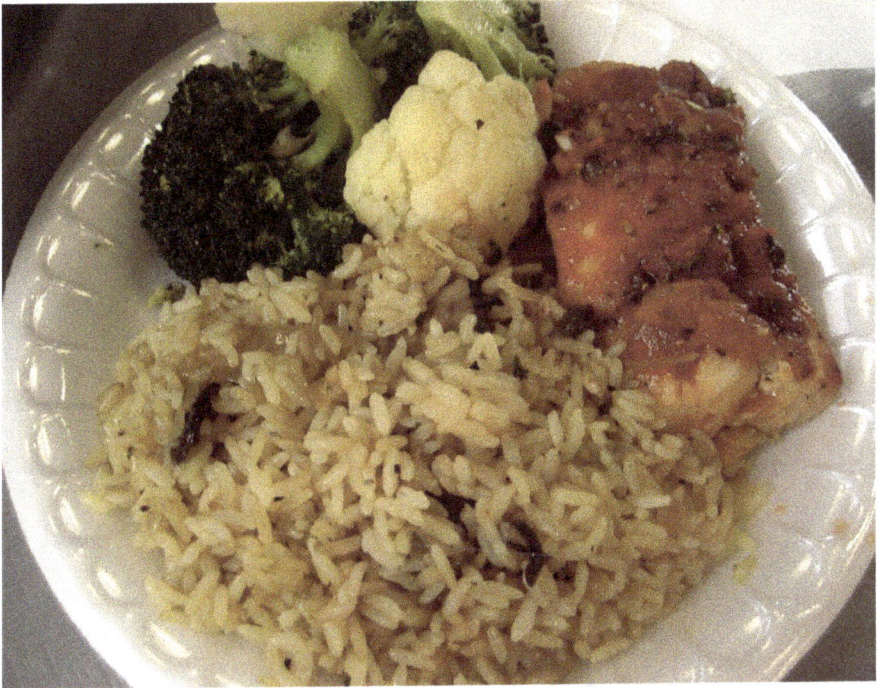

Cilantro Sea Bass

Prep time: 10 minutes I **Cooking time:** 15 minutes I **Servings:** 4

Ingredients:

- 1 tablespoon balsamic vinegar
- 1 tablespoon ginger, grated
- 2 tablespoons olive oil
- Black pepper to the taste
- 4 sea bass fillets, boneless
- 1 tablespoon cilantro, chopped

Directions:

1. Heat up a pan with the oil over medium heat, add the fish and cook for 5 minutes on each side.
2. Add the rest of the ingredients, cook everything for 5 minutes more, divide everything between plates and serve.

Nutrition info per serving: calories 267, fat 11.2, fiber 5.2, carbs 14.3, protein 14.3

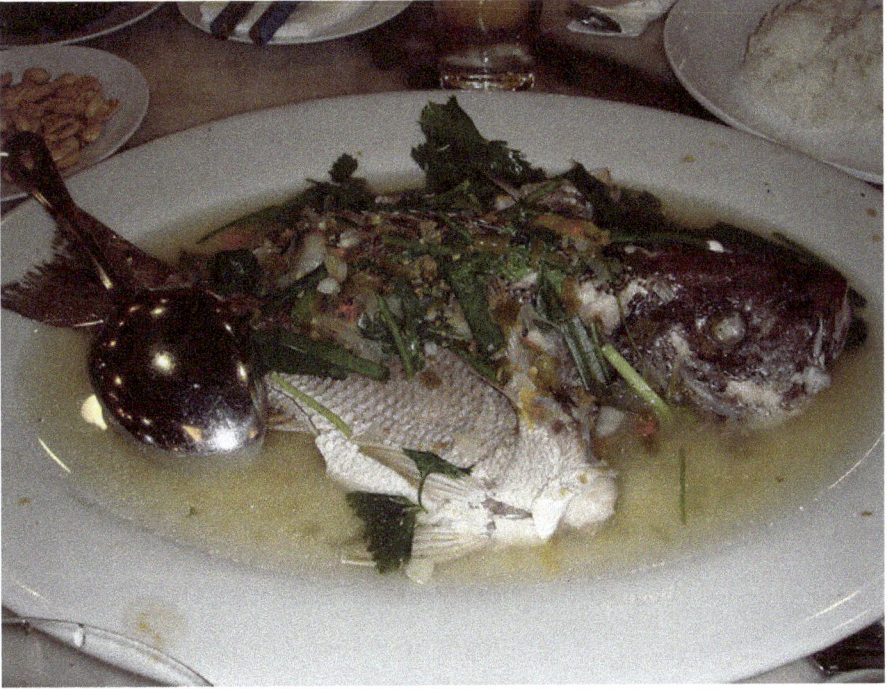

Balsamic Salmon and Beans

Prep time: 10 minutes I **Cooking time:** 20 minutes I **Servings:** 4

Ingredients:

- 2 tablespoons olive oil
- 1 cup chicken stock
- 4 salmon fillets, boneless
- 2 garlic cloves, minced
- 1 tablespoon ginger, grated
- ½ pound green beans, trimmed and halved
- 2 teaspoons balsamic vinegar
- ¼ cup scallions, chopped

Directions:

1. Heat up a pan with the oil over medium heat, add the scallion and the garlic and sauté for 5 minutes.
2. Add the salmon and cook it for 5 minutes on each side.
3. Add the rest of the ingredients, cook everything for 5 minutes more, divide between plates and serve.

Nutrition info per serving: calories 220, fat 11.6, fiber 2, carbs 17.2, protein 9.3

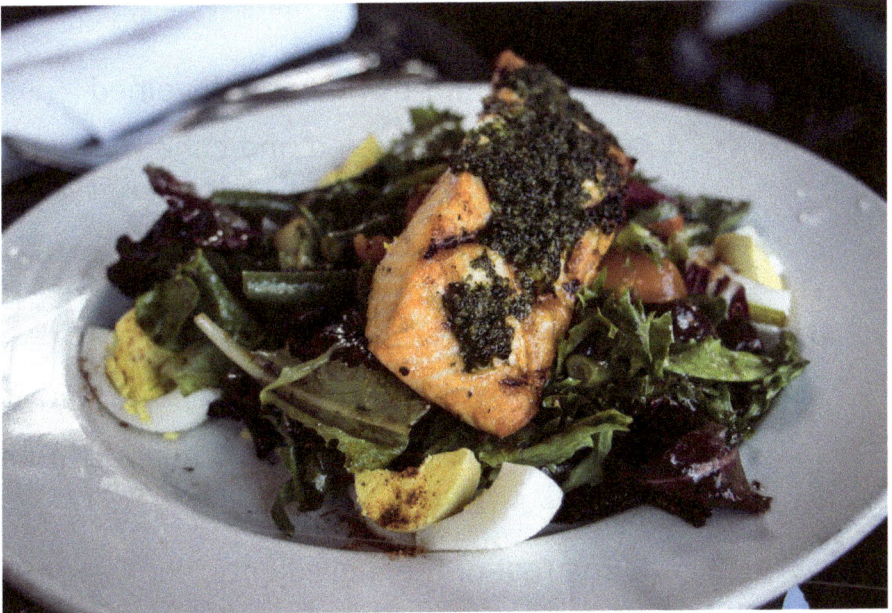

Parsley Shrimp Mix

Prep time: 10 minutes I **Cooking time:** 10 minutes I
Servings: 4

Ingredients:

- 1 tablespoon olive oil
- 1 pound shrimp, peeled and deveined
- 1 cup pineapple, peeled and cubed
- Juice of 1 lemon
- A bunch of parsley, chopped

Directions:

1. Heat up a pan with the oil over medium heat, add the shrimp and cook for 3 minutes on each side.
2. Add the rest of the ingredients, cook everything for 4 minutes more, divide into bowls and serve.

Nutrition info per serving: calories 254, fat 13.3, fiber 6, carbs 14.9, protein 11

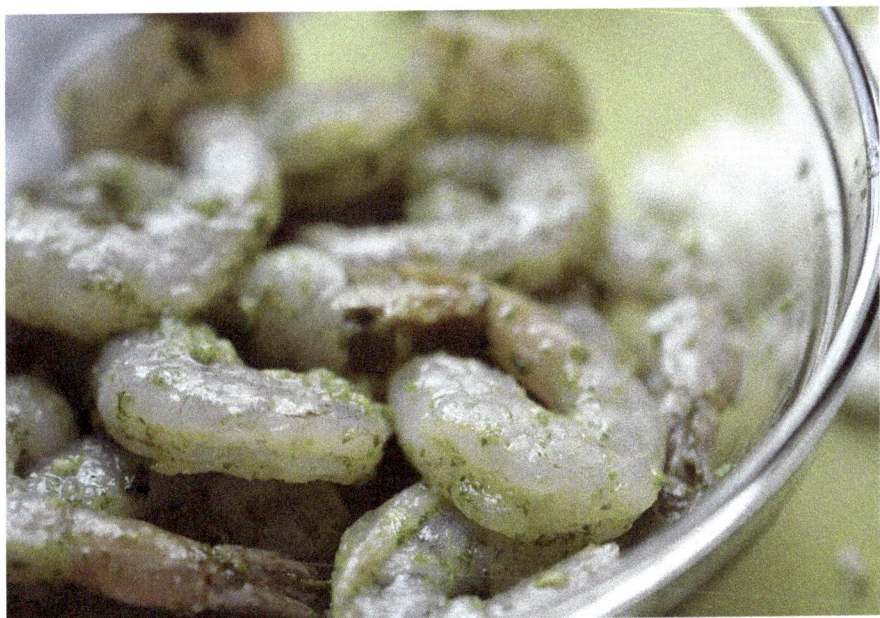

Chives Salmon and Olives

Prep time: 10 minutes I **Cooking time:** 20 minutes I
Servings: 4

Ingredients:

- 1 yellow onion, chopped
- 1 cup green olives, pitted and halved
- 1 teaspoon chili powder
- Black pepper to the taste
- 2 tablespoons olive oil
- ¼ cup veggie stock
- 4 salmon fillets, skinless and boneless
- 2 tablespoons chives, chopped

Directions:

1. Heat up a pan with the oil over medium-high heat, add the onion and sauté for 3 minutes.
2. Add the salmon and cook for 5 minutes on each side.

   Add the rest of the ingredients, cook the mix for 5 minutes more, divide between plates and serve.

Nutrition info per serving: calories 221, fat 12.1, fiber 5.4, carbs 8.5, protein 11.2

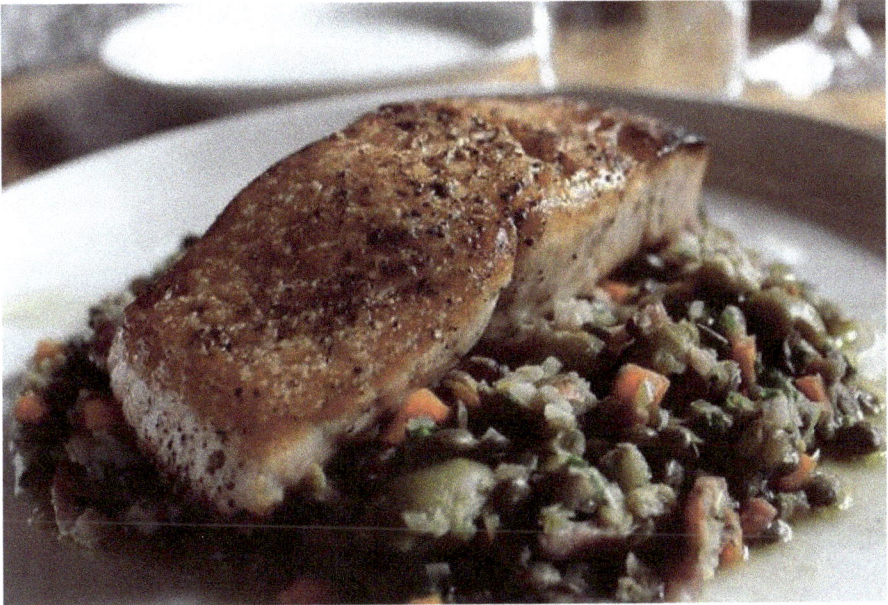

Lemon Salmon and Endives

Prep time: 5 minutes I **Cooking time:** 15 minutes I
Servings: 4

Ingredients:

- 4 medium salmon fillets, skinless and boneless
- 2 endives, shredded
- ½ cup veggie stock
- 2 tablespoons olive oil
- Black pepper to the taste
- 1 tablespoon lemon juice
- 1 tablespoon cilantro, chopped

Directions:

1. Heat up a pan with the oil over medium heat, add the endives and cook for 3 minutes.
2. Add the fish and brown it for 4 minutes on each side.
3. Add the rest of the ingredients, cook everything for 4 minutes more, divide between plates and serve.

Nutrition info per serving: calories 252, fat 9.3, fiber 4.2, carbs 12.3, protein 9

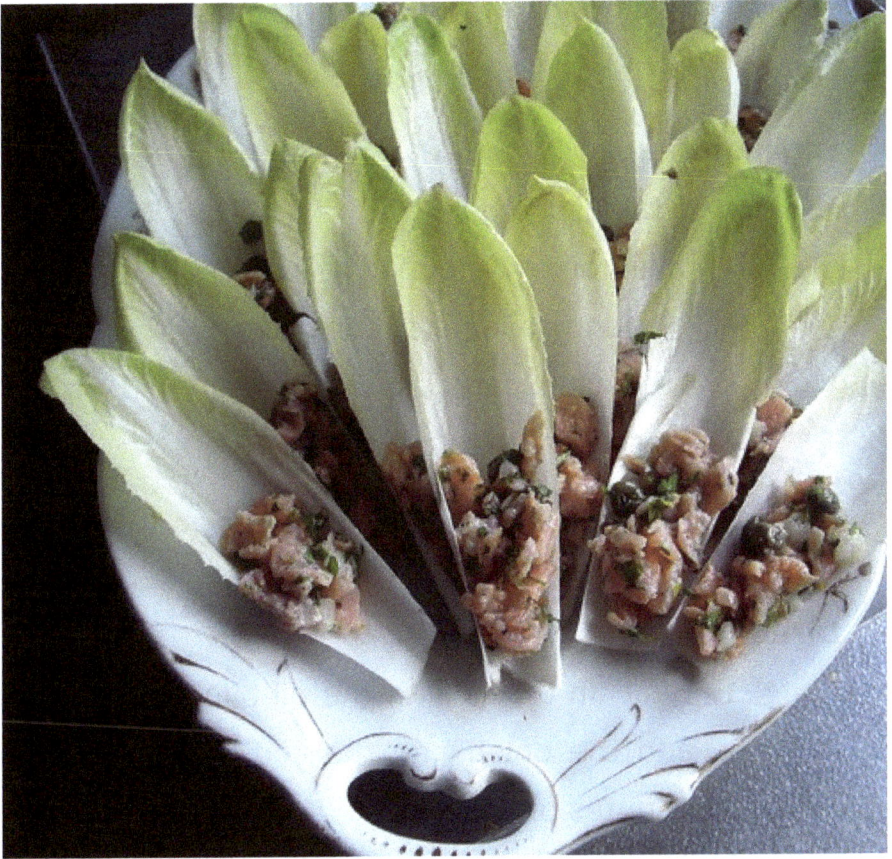

Coconut Cod and Asparagus

Prep time: 10 minutes I **Cooking time:** 14 minutes I
Servings: 4

Ingredients:

- 1 tablespoon olive oil
- 1 red onion, chopped
- 1 pound cod fillets, boneless
- 1 bunch asparagus, trimmed
- Black pepper to the taste
- 1 cup coconut cream
- 1 tablespoon chives, chopped

Directions:

1. Heat up a pan with the oil over medium heat, add the onion and the cod and cook it for 3 minutes on each side.
2. Add the rest of the ingredients, cook everything for 8 minutes more, divide between plates and serve.

Nutrition info per serving: calories 254, fat 12.1, fiber 5.4, carbs 4.2, protein 13.5

Cumin Shrimp

Prep time: 5 minutes I **Cooking time:** 8 minutes I
Servings: 4

Ingredients:

- 1 teaspoon garlic powder
- 1 teaspoon smoked paprika
- 1 teaspoon cumin, ground
- 1 teaspoon allspice, ground
- 2 tablespoons olive oil
- 2 pounds shrimp, peeled and deveined
- 1 tablespoon chives, chopped

Directions:

1. Heat up a pan with the oil over medium heat, add the shrimp, garlic powder and the other ingredients, cook for 4 minutes on each side, divide into bowls and serve.

Nutrition info per serving: calories 212, fat 9.6, fiber 5.3, carbs 12.7, protein 15.4

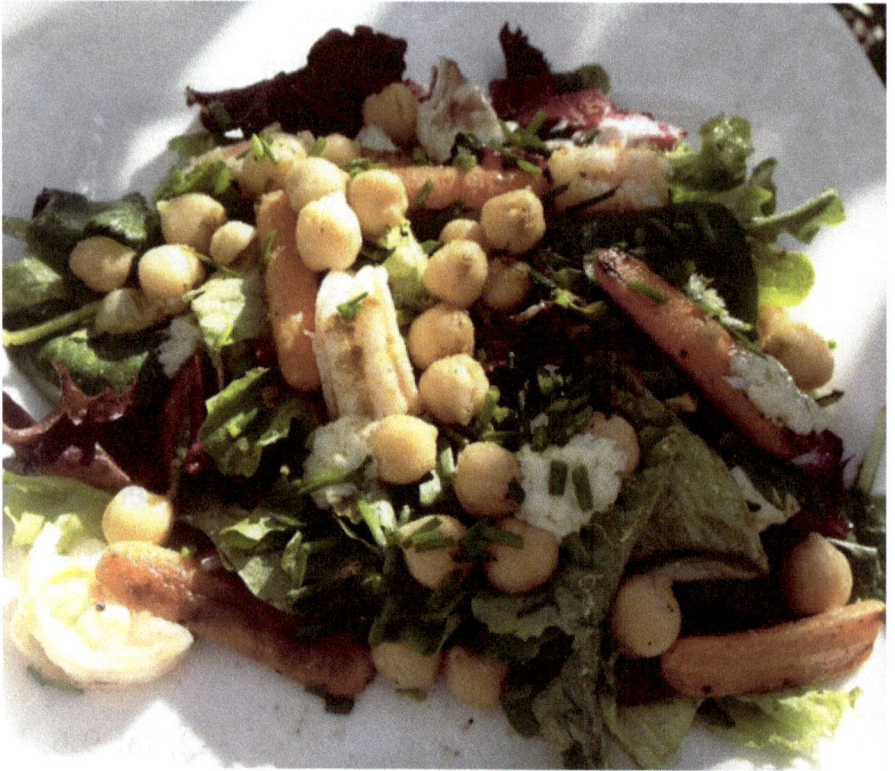

Sea Bass Mix

Prep time: 10 minutes I **Cooking time:** 30 minutes I
Servings: 4

Ingredients:

- 2 tablespoons olive oil
- 2 pounds sea bass fillets, skinless and boneless
- Black pepper to the taste
- 2 cups cherry tomatoes, halved
- 1 tablespoon chives, chopped
- 1 tablespoon lemon zest, grated
- ¼ cup lemon juice

Directions:

1. Grease a roasting pan with the oil and arrange the fish inside.
2. Add the tomatoes and the other ingredients, introduce the pan in the oven and bake at 380 degrees F for 30 minutes.
3. Divide everything between plates and serve.

Nutrition info per serving: calories 272, fat 6.9, fiber 6.2, carbs 18.4, protein 9

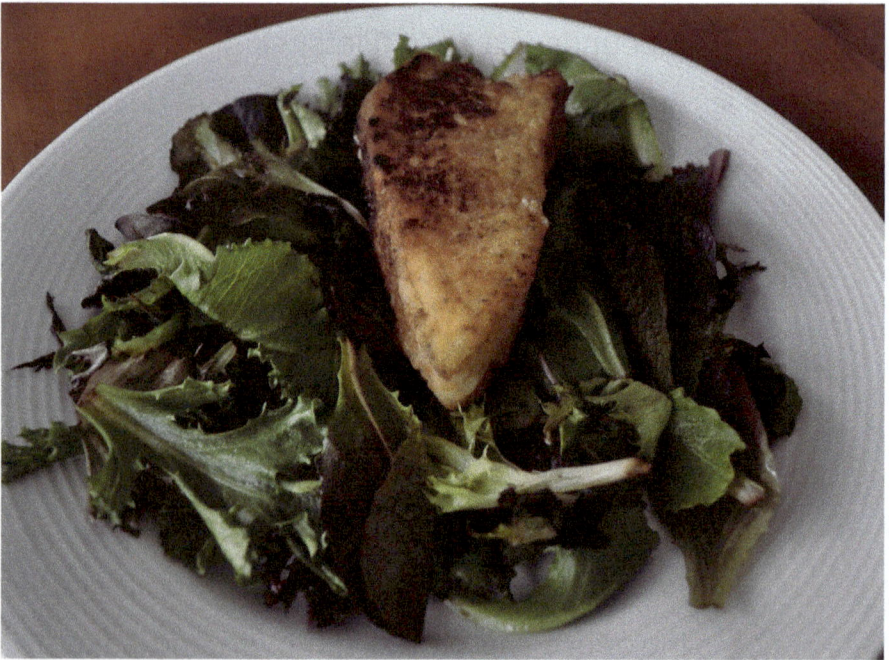

Oregano Shrimp

Prep time: 10 minutes I **Cooking time:** 12 minutes I
Servings: 4

Ingredients:

- 1 pound shrimp, deveined and peeled
- 1 tablespoon olive oil
- Juice of 1 lime
- 1 cup black beans, cooked
- 1 shallot, chopped
- 1 tablespoon oregano, chopped
- 2 garlic cloves, chopped
- Black pepper to the taste

Directions:

1. Heat up a pan with the oil over medium-high heat, add the shallot and the garlic, stir and cook for 3 minutes.
2. Add the shrimp and cook for 2 minutes on each side.
3. Add the beans and the other ingredients, cook everything over medium heat for 5 minutes more, divide into bowls and serve.

Nutrition info per serving: calories 253, fat 11.6, fiber 6, carbs 14.5, protein 13.5

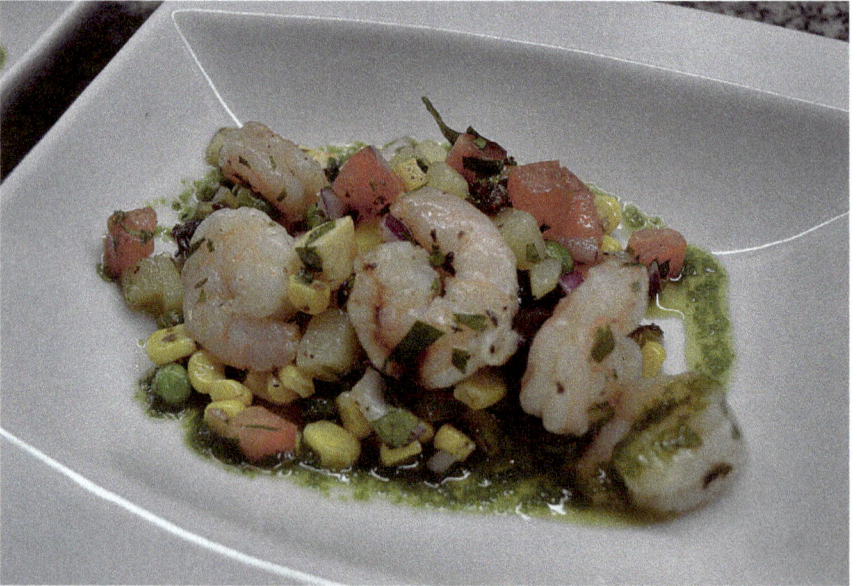

Shrimp and Shallots

Prep time: 5 minutes I **Cooking time:** 8 minutes I
Servings: 4

Ingredients:

- 1 pound shrimp, peeled and deveined
- 2 shallots, chopped
- 1 tablespoon olive oil
- 1 tablespoon chives, chopped
- 2 teaspoons prepared horseradish
- ¼ cup coconut cream
- Black pepper to the taste

Directions:

1. Heat up a pan with the oil over medium heat, add the shallots and the horseradish, stir and sauté for 2 minutes.
2. Add the shrimp and the other ingredients, toss, cook for 6 minutes more, divide between plates and serve.

Nutrition info per serving: calories 233, fat 6, fiber 5, carbs 11.9, protein 5.4

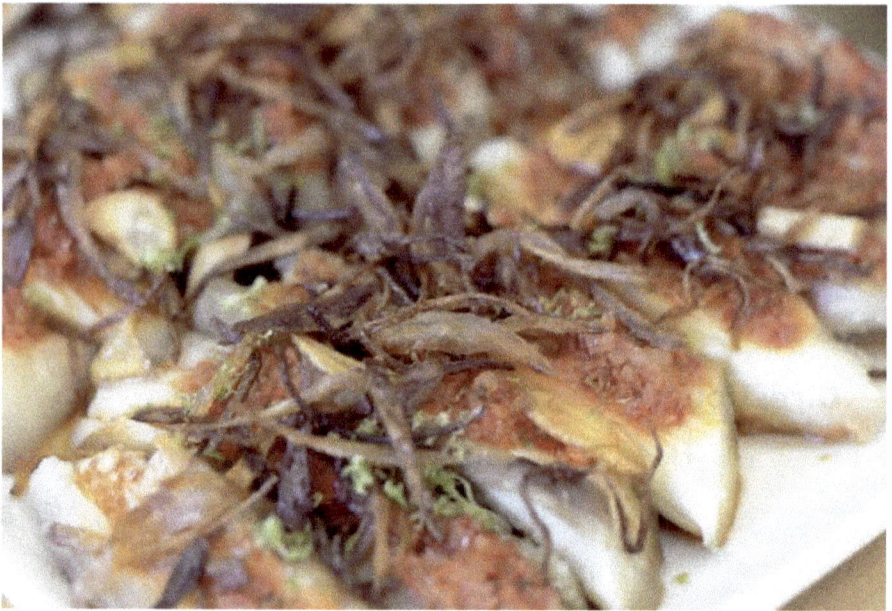

Shrimp and Capers Salad

Prep time: 4 minutes I **Cooking time:** 0 minutes I
Servings: 4

Ingredients:

- 1 pound shrimp, cooked, peeled and deveined
- 1 tablespoon tarragon, chopped
- 1 tablespoon capers, drained
- 2 tablespoons olive oil
- Black pepper to the taste
- 2 cups baby spinach
- 1 tablespoon balsamic vinegar
- 1 small red onion, sliced
- 2 tablespoons lemon juice

Directions:

1. In a bowl, combine the shrimp with the tarragon and the other ingredients, toss and serve.

Nutrition info per serving: calories 258, fat 12.4, fiber 6, carbs 6.7, protein 13.3

Cheesy Cod Mix

Prep time: 10 minutes I **Cooking time:** 20 minutes I **Servings:** 4

Ingredients:

- 4 cod fillets, boneless
- ½ cup parmesan cheese, shredded
- 3 garlic cloves, minced
- 1 tablespoon olive oil
- 1 tablespoon lemon juice
- ½ cup green onion, chopped

Directions:

1. Heat up a pan with the oil over medium heat, add the garlic and the green onions, toss and sauté for 5 minutes.
2. Add the fish and cook it for 4 minutes on each side.
3. Add the lemon juice, sprinkle the parmesan on top, cook everything for 2 minutes more, divide between plates and serve.

Nutrition info per serving: calories 275, fat 22.1, fiber 5, carbs 18.2, protein 12

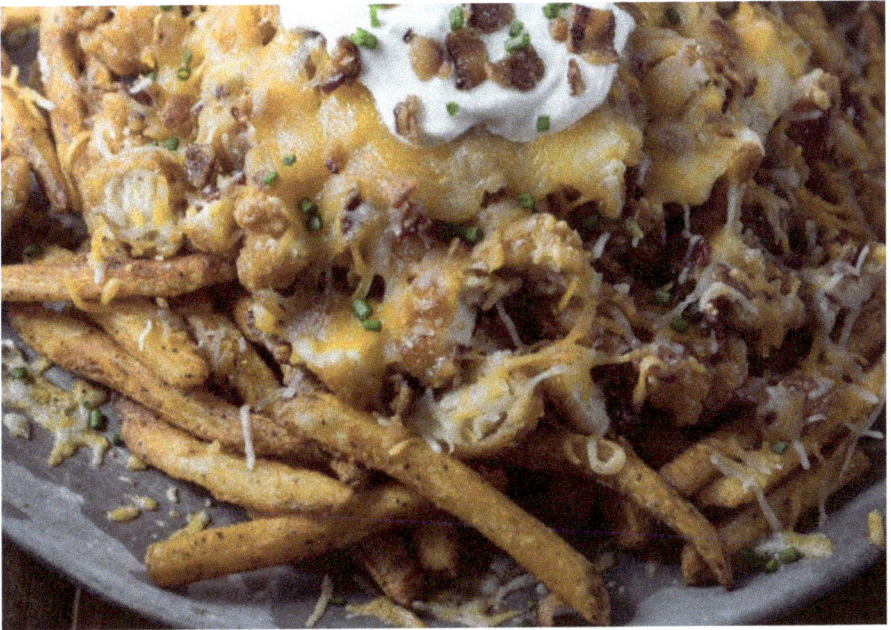

Lemony Tilapia Mix

Prep time: 10 minutes I **Cooking time:** 15 minutes I
Servings: 4

Ingredients:

- 4 tilapia fillets, boneless
- 2 tablespoons olive oil
- 1 tablespoon lemon juice
- 2 teaspoons lemon zest, grated
- 2 red onions, roughly chopped
- 3 tablespoons chives, chopped

Directions:

1. Heat up a pan with the oil over medium heat, add the onions, lemon zest and lemon juice, toss and sauté for 5 minutes.
2. Add the fish and the chives, cook for 5 minutes on each side, divide between plates and serve.

Nutrition info per serving: calories 254, fat 18.2, fiber 5.4, carbs 11.7, protein 4.5

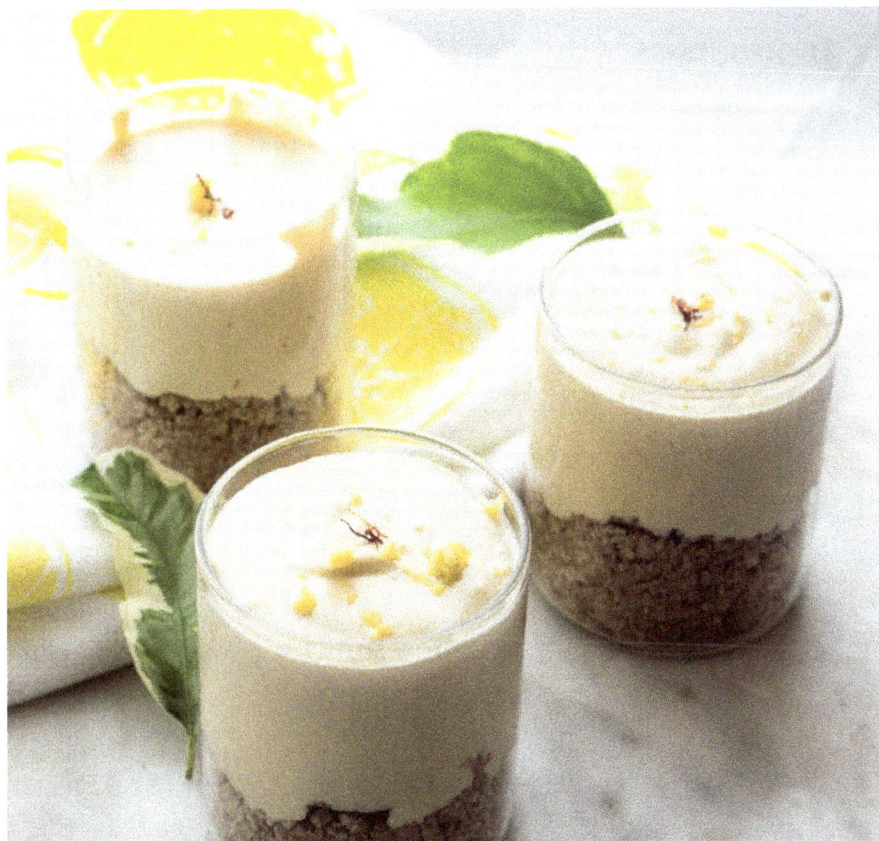

Trout and Avocado Salad

Prep time: 6 minutes I **Cooking time:** 0 minutes I
Servings: 4

Ingredients:

- 4 ounces smoked trout, skinless, boneless and cubed
- 1 tablespoon lime juice
- 1/3 cup yogurt
- 2 avocados, peeled, pitted and cubed
- 3 tablespoons chives, chopped
- Black pepper to the taste
- 1 tablespoon olive oil

Directions:

1. In a bowl, combine the trout with the avocados and the other ingredients, toss, and serve.

Nutrition info per serving: calories 244, fat 9.45, fiber 5.6, carbs 8.5, protein 15

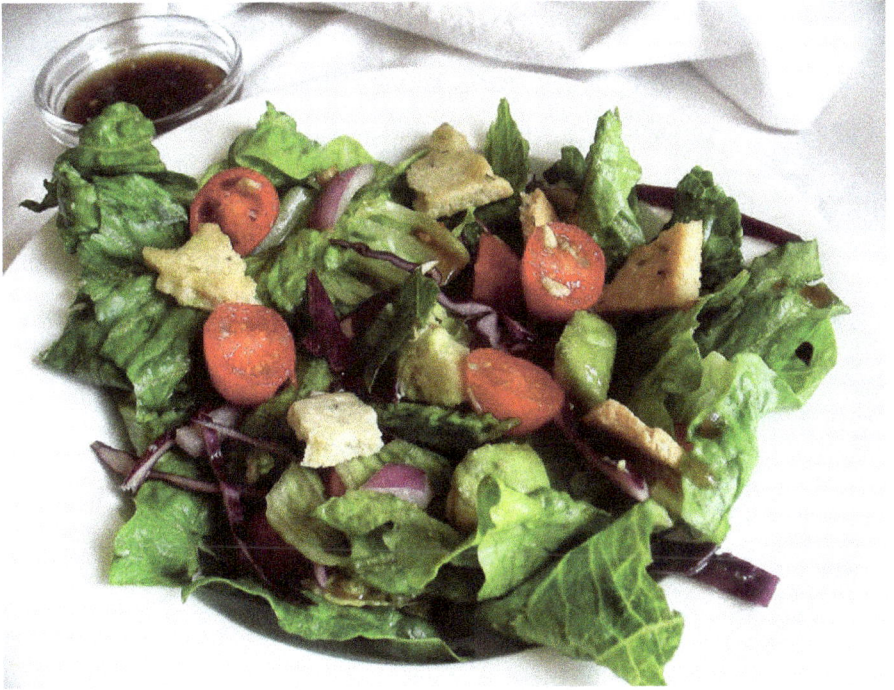

Garlic Trout

Prep time: 5 minutes I **Cooking time:** 15 minutes I
Servings: 4

Ingredients:

- 3 tablespoons balsamic vinegar
- 2 tablespoons olive oil
- 4 trout fillets, boneless
- 3 tablespoons parsley, finely chopped
- 2 garlic cloves, minced

Directions:

1. Heat up a pan with the oil over medium heat, add the trout and cook for 6 minutes on each side.
2. Add the rest of the ingredients, cook for 3 minutes more, divide between plates and serve with a side salad.

Nutrition info per serving: calories 314, fat 14.3, fiber 8.2, carbs 14.8, protein 11.2

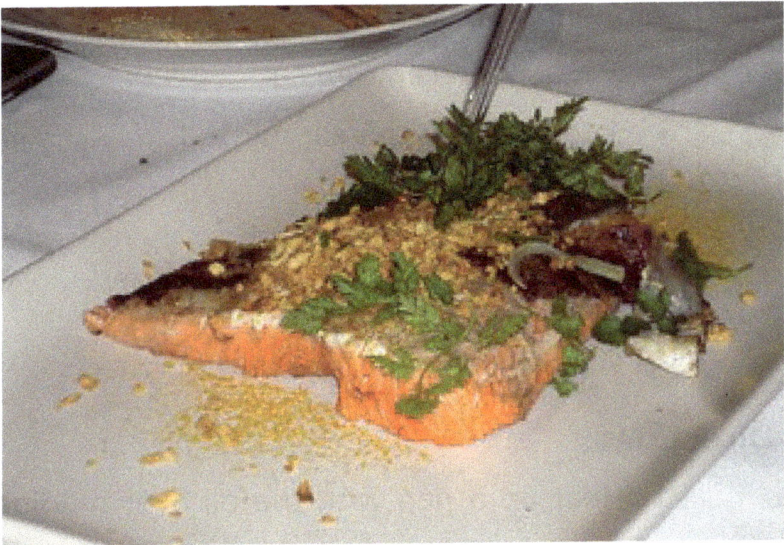

Parsley Salmon

Prep time: 5 minutes I **Cooking time:** 12 minutes I
Servings: 4

Ingredients:

- 2 spring onions, chopped
- 2 teaspoons lime juice
- 1 tablespoon chives, minced
- 1 tablespoon olive oil
- 4 salmon fillets, boneless
- Black pepper to the taste
- 2 tablespoons parsley, chopped

Directions:

1. Heat up a pan with the oil over medium heat, add the spring onions, stir and sauté for 2 minutes.
2. Add the salmon and the other ingredients, cook for 5 minutes on each side, divide between plates and serve.

Nutrition info per serving: calories 290, fat 14.4, fiber 5.6, carbs 15.6, protein 9.5

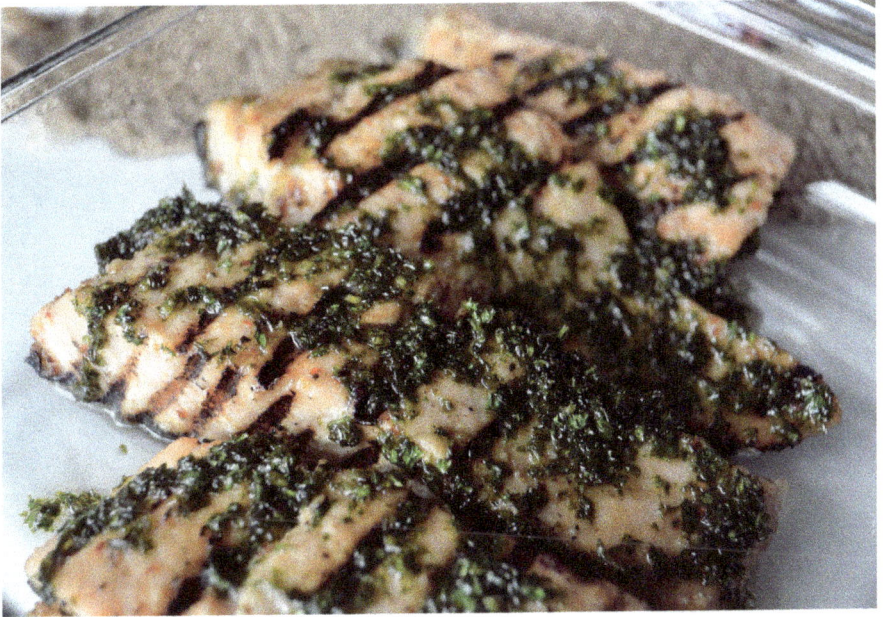

Trout and Arugula Salad

Prep time: 5 minutes I **Cooking time:** 0 minutes I
Servings: 4

Ingredients:

- 2 tablespoons olive oil
- ½ cup kalamata olives, pitted and minced
- Black pepper to the taste
- 1 pound smoked trout, boneless, skinless and cubed
- ½ teaspoon lemon zest, grated
- 1 tablespoon lemon juice
- 1 cup cherry tomatoes, halved
- ½ red onion, sliced
- 2 cups baby arugula

Directions:

1. In a bowl, combine smoked trout with the olives, black pepper and the other ingredients, toss and serve.

Nutrition info per serving: calories 282, fat 13.4, fiber 5.3, carbs 11.6, protein 5.6

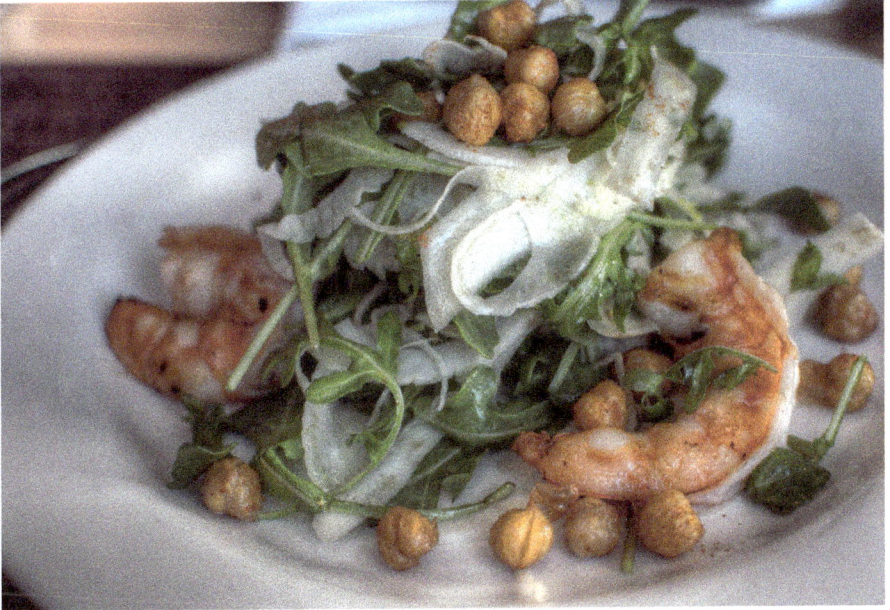

Saffron Paprika Salmon

Prep time: 10 minutes I **Cooking time:** 12 minutes I
Servings: 4

Ingredients:

- Black pepper to the taste
- ½ teaspoon sweet paprika
- 4 salmon fillets, boneless
- 3 tablespoons olive oil
- 1 yellow onion, chopped
- 2 garlic cloves, minced
- ¼ teaspoon saffron powder

Directions:

1. Heat up a pan with the oil over medium-high heat, add the onion and the garlic, toss and sauté for 2 minutes.
2. Add the salmon and the other ingredients, cook for 5 minutes on each side, divide between plates and serve.

Nutrition info per serving: calories 339, fat 21.6, fiber 0.7, carbs 3.2, protein 35

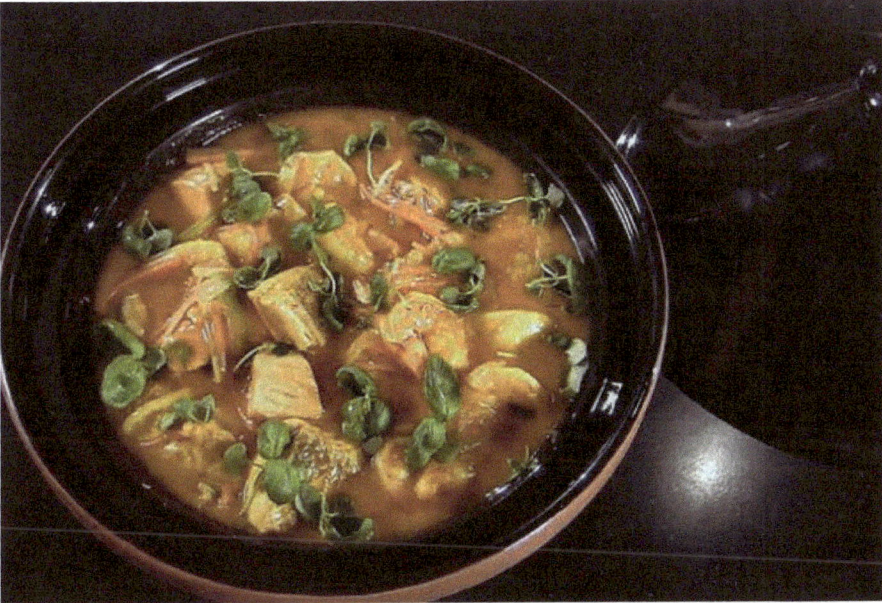

Shrimp and Basil Salad

Prep time: 10 minutes I **Cooking time:** 0 minutes I
Servings: 4

Ingredients:

- ¼ cup basil, chopped
- 2 cups watermelon, peeled and cubed
- 2 tablespoons balsamic vinegar
- 2 tablespoons olive oil
- 1 pound shrimp, peeled, deveined and cooked
- Black pepper to the taste
- 1 tablespoon parsley, chopped

Directions:

1. In a bowl, combine the shrimp with the watermelon and the other ingredients, toss and serve.

Nutrition info per serving: calories 220, fat 9, fiber 0.4, carbs 7.6, protein 26.4

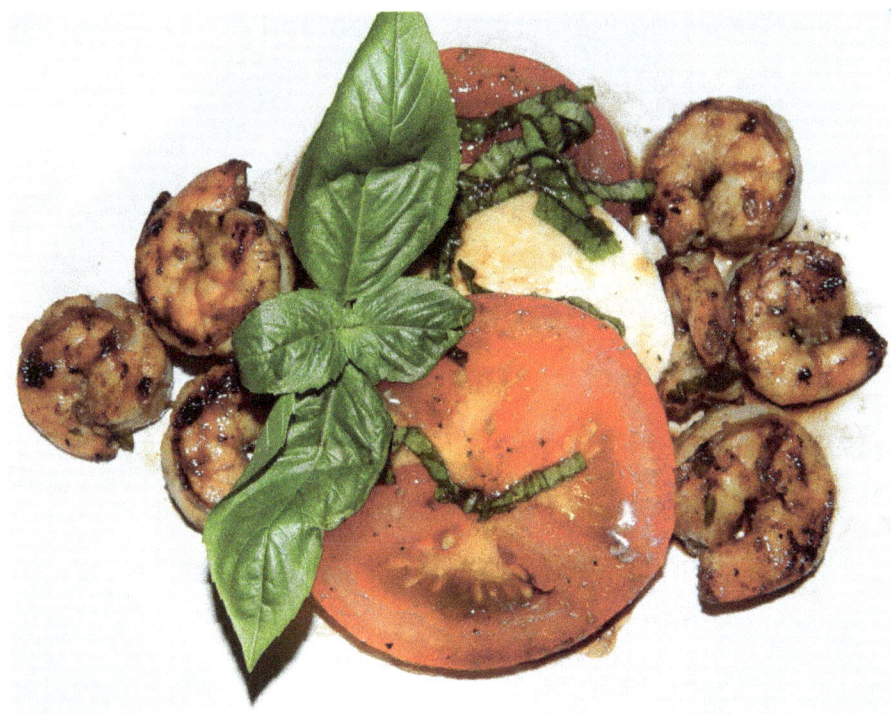

Shrimp and Quinoa Salad

Prep time: 5 minutes I **Cooking time:** 8 minutes I
Servings: 4

Ingredients:

- 1 pound shrimp, peeled and deveined
- 1 cup quinoa, cooked
- Black pepper to the taste
- 1 tablespoon olive oil
- 1 tablespoon oregano, chopped
- 1 red onion, chopped
- Juice of 1 lemon

Directions:

1. Heat up a pan with the oil over medium-high heat, add the onion, stir and sauté for 2 minutes.
2. Add the shrimp, toss and cook for 5 minutes.
3. Add the rest of the ingredients, toss, divide everything into bowls and serve.

Nutrition info per serving: calories 336, fat 8.2, fiber 4.1, carbs 32.3, protein 32.3

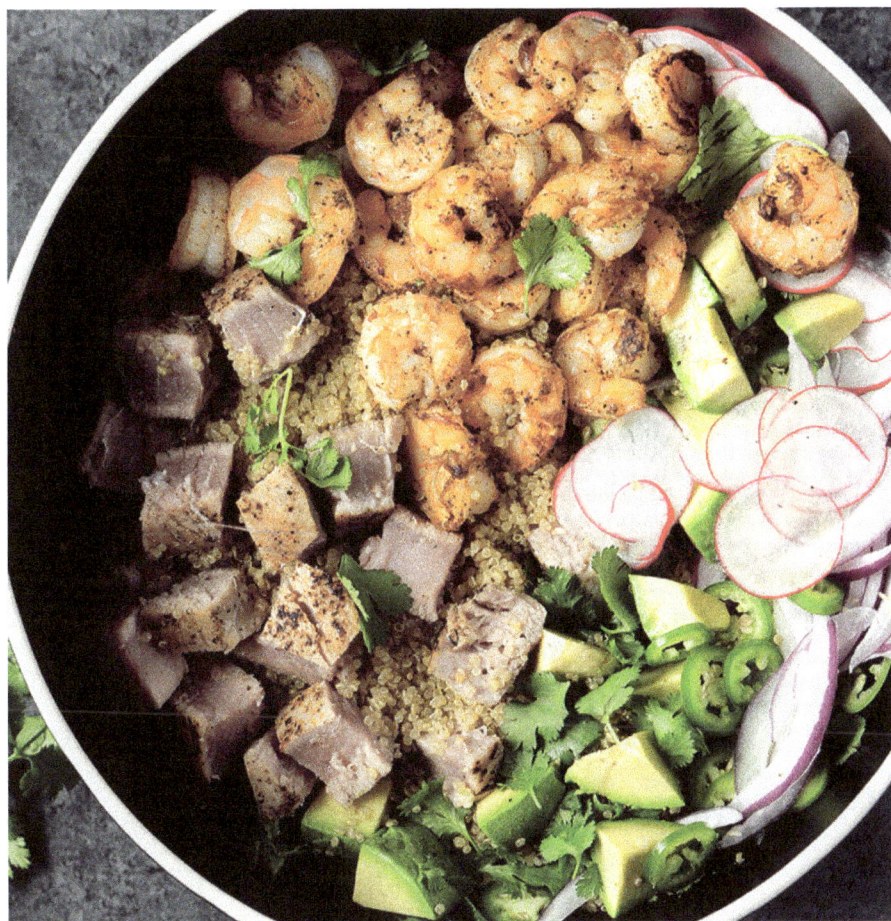

Crab and Cherry Tomato Salad

Prep time: 10 minutes I **Cooking time:** 0 minutes I
Servings: 4

Ingredients:

- 1 tablespoon olive oil
- 2 cups crab meat
- Black pepper to the taste
- 1 cup cherry tomatoes, halved
- 1 shallot, chopped
- 1 tablespoon lemon juice
- 1/3 cup cilantro, chopped

Directions:

1. In a bowl, combine the crab with the tomatoes and the other ingredients, toss and serve.

Nutrition info per serving: calories 54, fat 3.9, fiber 0.6, carbs 2.6, protein 2.3

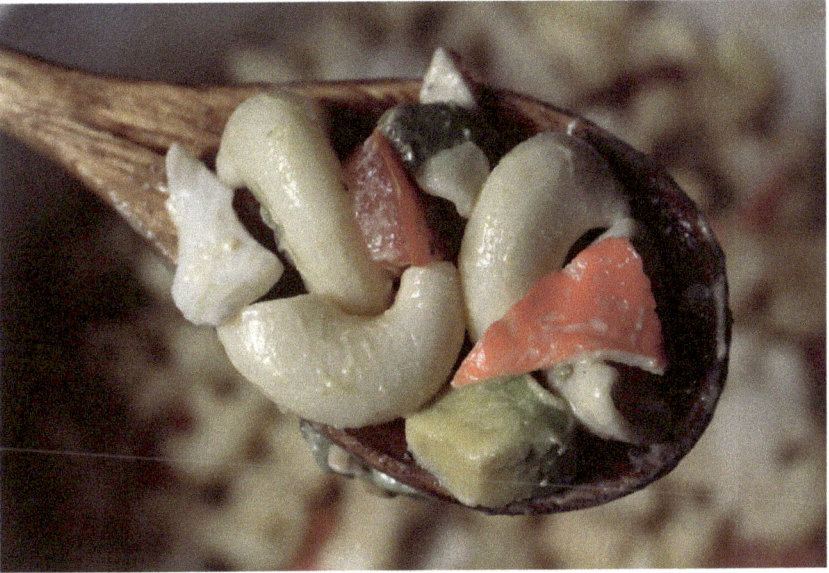

Scallops and Scallions

Prep time: 4 minutes I **Cooking time:** 6 minutes I

Servings: 4

Ingredients:

- 12 ounces sea scallops
- 2 tablespoons olive oil
- 2 garlic cloves, minced
- 1 tablespoon balsamic vinegar
- 1 cup scallions, sliced
- 2 tablespoons cilantro, chopped

Directions:

1. Heat up a pan with the oil over medium heat, add the scallions and the garlic and sauté for 2 minutes.
2. Add the scallops and the other ingredients, cook them for 2 minutes on each side, divide between plates and serve.

Nutrition info per serving: calories 146, fat 7.7, fiber 0.7, carbs 4.4, protein 14.8

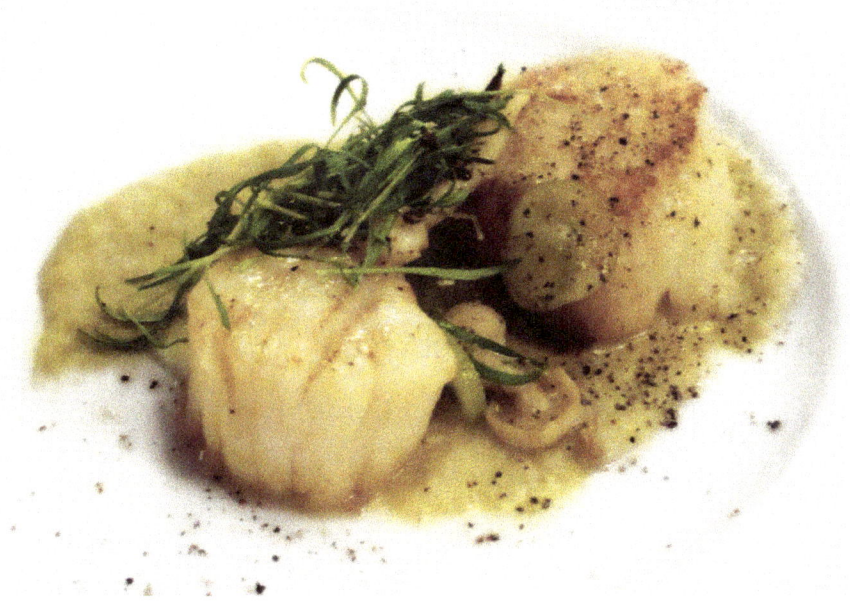

Dill Flounder Mix

Prep time: 10 minutes I **Cooking time:** 20 minutes I
Servings: 4

Ingredients:

- 2 tablespoon olive oil
- 1 red onion, chopped
- Black pepper to the taste
- ½ cup veggie stock
- 4 flounder fillets, boneless
- ½ cup coconut cream
- 1 tablespoon dill, chopped

Directions:

1. Heat up a pan with the oil over medium heat, add the onion, stir and sauté for 5 minutes.
2. Add the fish and cook it for 4 minutes on each side.
3. Add the rest of the ingredients, cook for 7 minutes more, divide between plates and serve.

Nutrition info per serving: calories 232, fat 12.3, fiber 4, carbs 8.7, protein 12

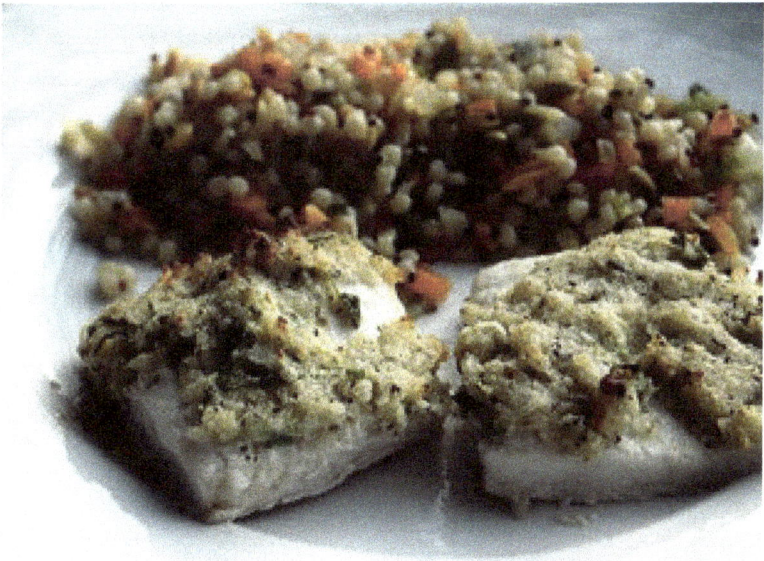

Salmon and Mango

Prep time: 5 minutes I **Cooking time:** 0 minutes I
Servings: 4

Ingredients:

- 1 pound smoked salmon, boneless, skinless and flaked
- Black pepper to the taste
- 1 red onion, chopped
- 1 mango, peeled, seedless and chopped
- 2 jalapeno peppers, chopped
- ¼ cup parsley, chopped
- 3 tablespoons lime juice
- 1 tablespoon olive oil

Directions:

2. In a bowl, mix the salmon with the black pepper and the other ingredients, toss and serve.

Nutrition info per serving: calories 323, fat 14.2, fiber 4, carbs 8.5, protein 20.4

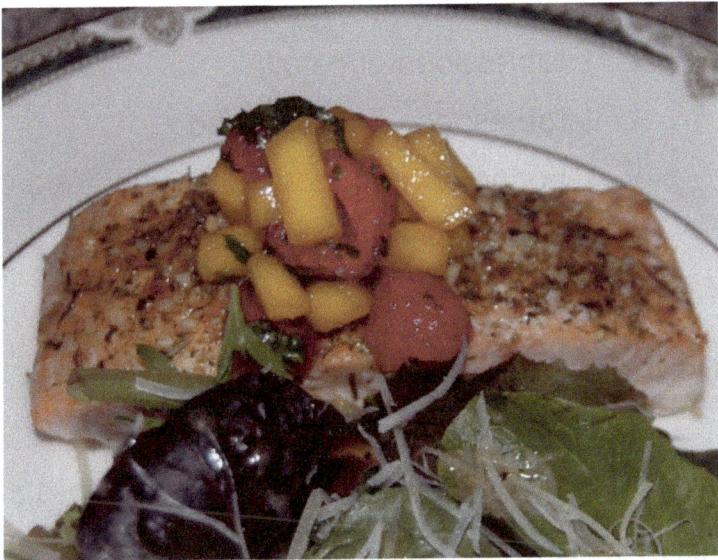

Shrimp and Radish Mix

Prep time: 5 minutes I **Cooking time:** 0 minutes I
Servings: 4

Ingredients:

- 2 teaspoons lemon juice
- 1 tablespoon olive oil
- 1 tablespoon dill, chopped
- 1 pound shrimp, cooked, peeled and deveined
- Black pepper to the taste
- 1 cup radishes, cubed

Directions:

1. In a bowl, combine the shrimp with the lemon juice and the other ingredients, toss and serve.

Nutrition info per serving: calories 292, fat 13, fiber 4.4, carbs 8, protein 16.4

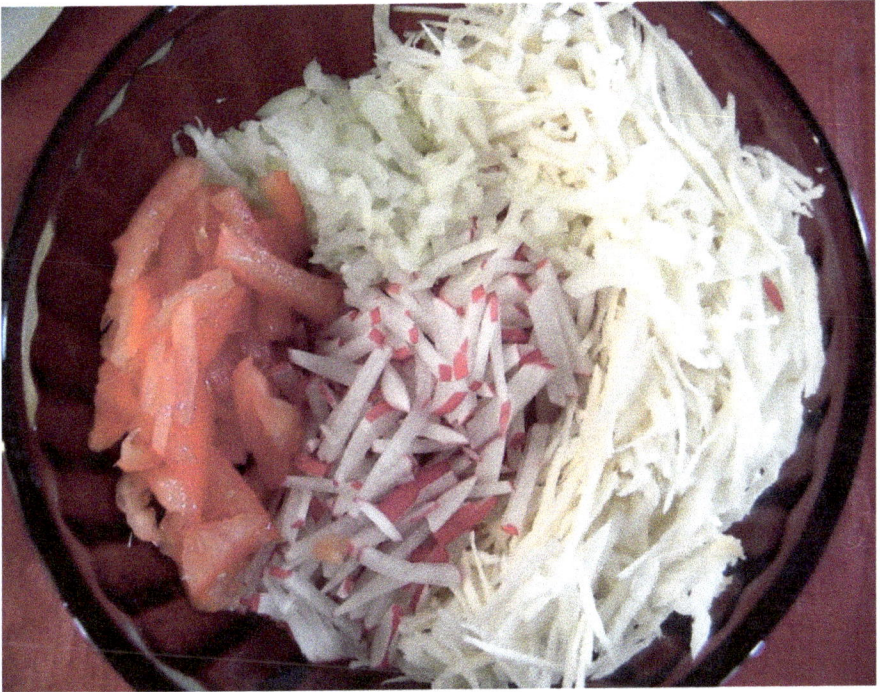

Cheesy Salmon Spread

Prep time: 4 minutes I **Cooking time:** 0 minutes I
Servings: 6

Ingredients:

- 6 ounces smoked salmon, boneless, skinless
  and shredded
- 2 tablespoons non-fat yogurt
- 3 teaspoons lemon juice
- 2 spring onions, chopped
- 8 ounces cream cheese
- ¼ cup cilantro, chopped

Directions:

1. In a bowl, mix the salmon with the yogurt and
   the other ingredients, whisk and serve cold.

Nutrition info per serving: calories 272, fat 15.2, fiber
4.3, carbs 16.8, protein 9.9

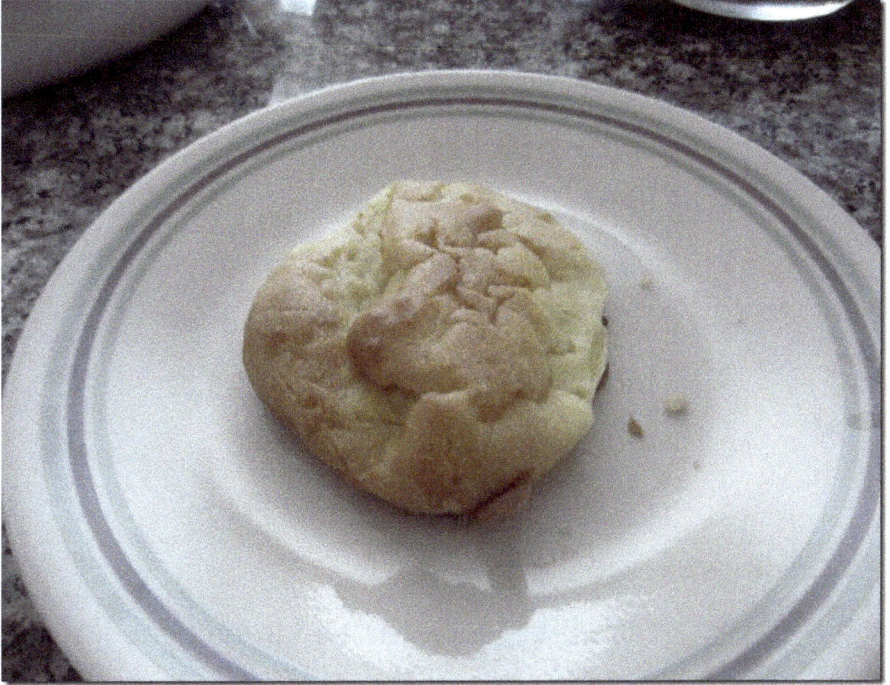

Shrimp with Artichokes and Tomatoes

Prep time: 4 minutes I **Cooking time:** 8 minutes I
Servings: 4

Ingredients:

- 2 green onions, chopped
- 1 cup artichokes, quartered
- 2 tablespoons cilantro, chopped
- 1 pound shrimp, peeled and deveined
- 1 cup cherry tomatoes, cubed
- 1 tablespoon olive oil
- 1 tablespoon balsamic vinegar
- A pinch of salt and black pepper

Directions:

1. Heat up a pan with the oil over medium heat, add the onions and the artichokes, toss and cook for 2 minutes.
2. Add the shrimp, toss and cook over medium heat for 6 minutes.
3. Divide everything into bowls and serve.

Nutrition info per serving: calories 260, fat 8.23, fiber 3.8, carbs 14.3, protein 12.4

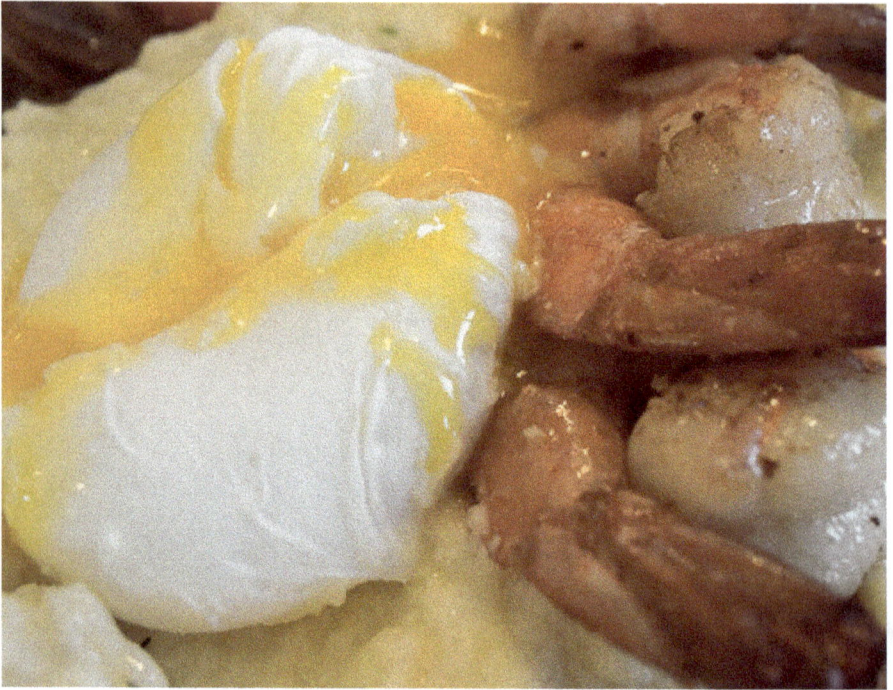

Shrimp and Sauce

Prep time: 5 minutes I **Cooking time:** 8 minutes I

Servings: 4

Ingredients:

- 1 pound shrimp, peeled and deveined
- 2 tablespoons olive oil
- Zest of 1 lemon, grated
- Juice of ½ lemon
- 1 tablespoon chives, chopped

Directions:

1. Heat up a pan with the oil over medium-high heat, add the lemon zest, lemon juice and the cilantro, toss and cook for 2 minutes.
2. Add the shrimp, cook everything for 6 minutes more, divide between plates and serve.

Nutrition info per serving: calories 195, fat 8.9, fiber 0, carbs 1.8, protein 25.9

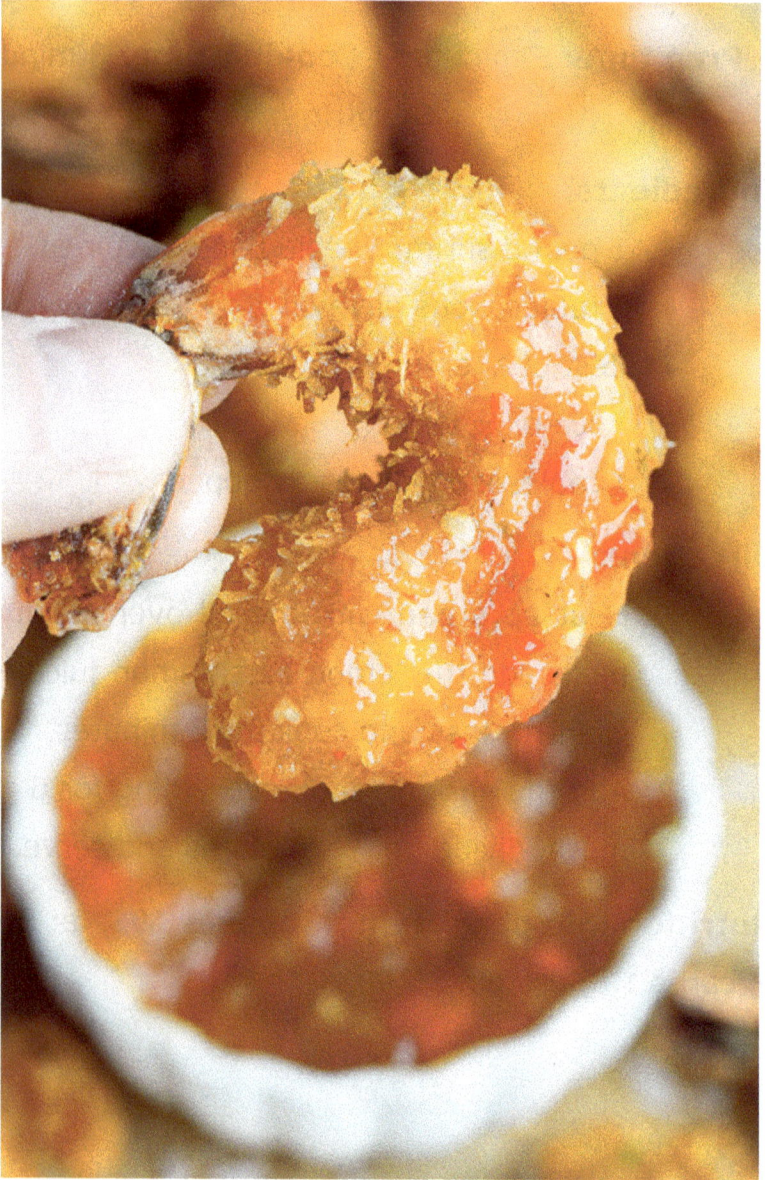

Oregano Tuna and Orange

Prep time: 5 minutes I **Cooking time:** 12 minutes I
Servings: 4

Ingredients:

- 4 tuna fillets, boneless
- Black pepper to the taste
- 2 tablespoons olive oil
- 2 shallots, chopped
- 3 tablespoons orange juice
- 1 orange, peeled and cut into segments
- 1 tablespoon oregano, chopped

Directions:

1. Heat up a pan with the oil over medium-high heat, add the shallots, stir and sauté for 2 minutes.
2. Add the tuna and the other ingredients, cook everything for 10 minutes more, divide between plates and serve.

Nutrition info per serving: calories 457, fat 38.2, fiber 1.6, carbs 8.2, protein 21.8

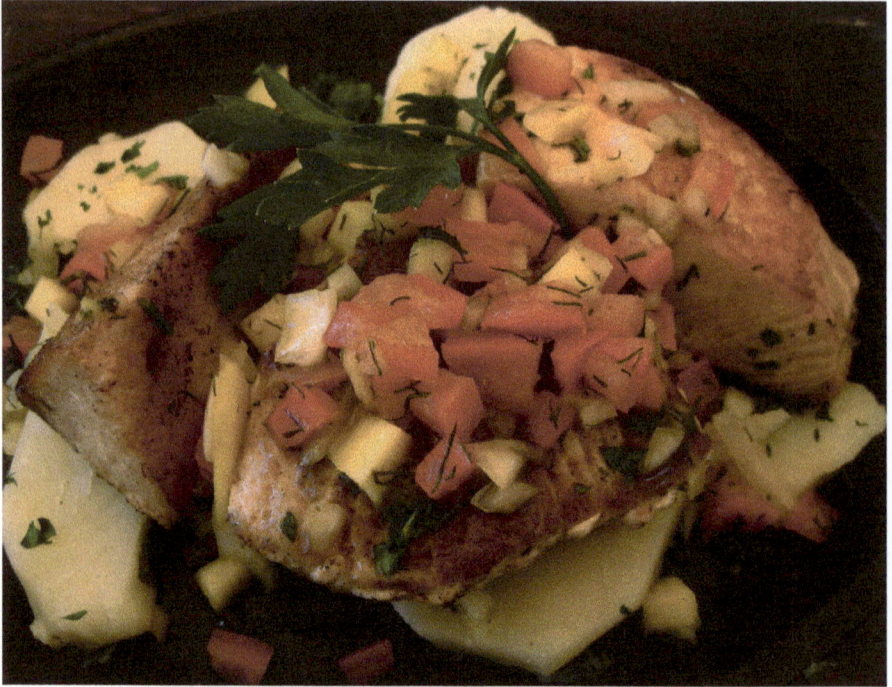

Fish Curry

Prep time: 10 minutes I **Cooking time:** 20 minutes I
Servings: 4

Ingredients:

- 1 pound salmon fillet, boneless and cubed
- 3 tablespoons red curry paste
- 1 red onion, chopped
- 1 teaspoon sweet paprika
- 1 cup coconut cream
- 1 tablespoon olive oil
- Black pepper to the taste
- ½ cup chicken stock
- 3 tablespoons basil, chopped

Directions:

1. Heat up a pan with the oil over medium-high heat, add the onion, paprika and the curry paste, toss and cook for 5 minutes.
2. Add the salmon and the other ingredients, toss gently, cook over medium heat for 15 minutes, divide into bowls and serve.

Nutrition info per serving: calories 377, fat 28.3, fiber 2.1, carbs 8.5, protein 23.9

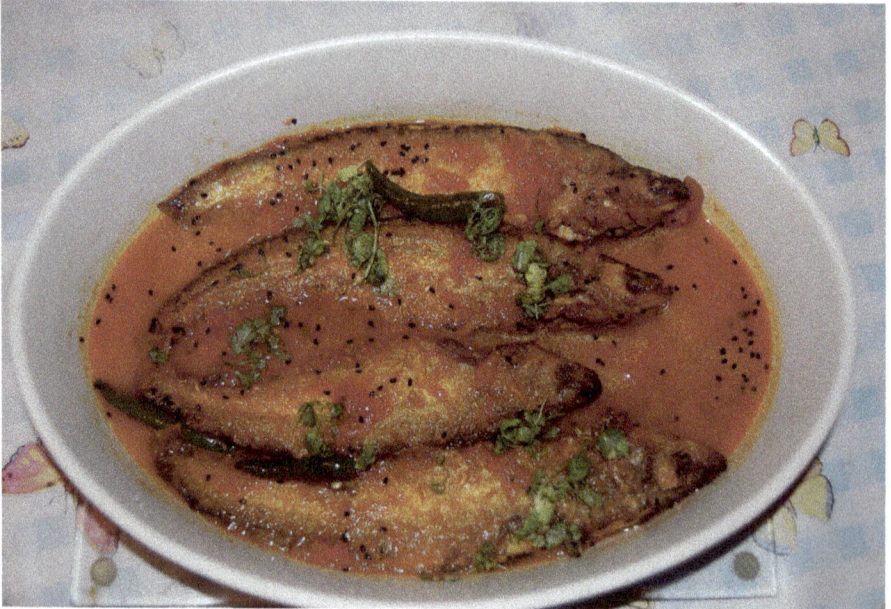

Salmon and Carrots Mix

Prep time: 10 minutes I **Cooking time:** 15 minutes I
Servings: 4

Ingredients:

- 4 salmon fillets, boneless
- 1 red onion, chopped
- 2 carrots, sliced
- 2 tablespoons olive oil
- 2 tablespoons balsamic vinegar
- Black pepper to the taste
- 2 tablespoons chives, chopped
- ¼ cup veggie stock

Directions:

1. Heat up a pan with the oil over medium heat, add the onion and the carrots, toss and sauté for 5 minutes.
2. Add the salmon and the other ingredients, cook everything for 10 minutes more, divide between plates and serve.

Nutrition info per serving: calories 322, fat 18, fiber 1.4, carbs 6, protein 35.2

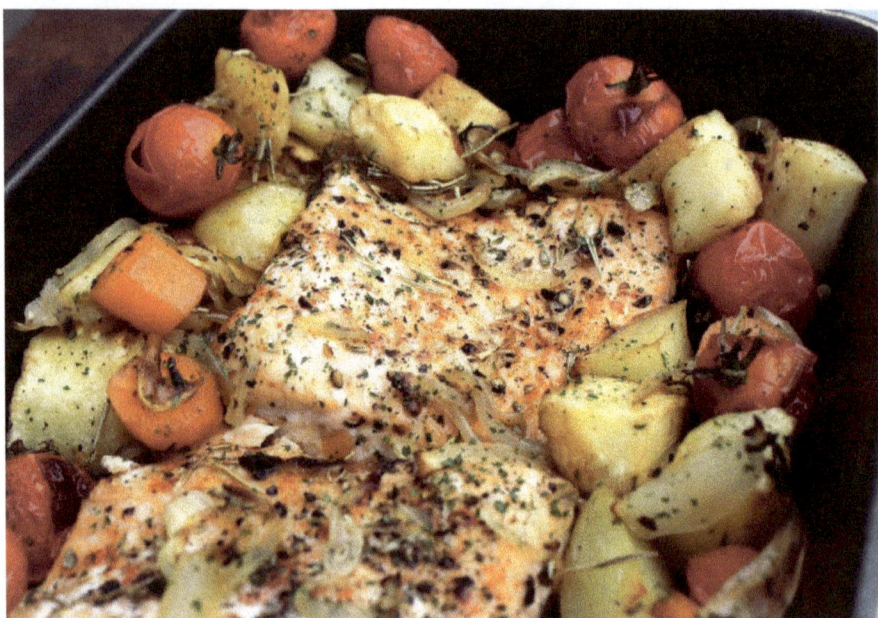

Thyme Shrimp

Prep time: 10 minutes I **Cooking time:** 10 minutes I
Servings: 4

Ingredients:

- 1 pound shrimp, peeled and deveined
- 2 tablespoons pine nuts
- 1 tablespoon lime juice
- 2 tablespoons olive oil
- 3 garlic cloves, minced
- Black pepper to the taste
- 1 tablespoon thyme, chopped
- 2 tablespoons chives, finely chopped

Directions:

1. Heat up a pan with the oil over medium-high heat, add the garlic, thyme, pine nuts and lime juice, toss and cook for 3 minutes.
2. Add the shrimp, black pepper and the chives, toss, cook for 7 minutes more, divide between plates and serve.

Nutrition info per serving: calories 290, fat 13, fiber 4.5, carbs 13.9, protein 10

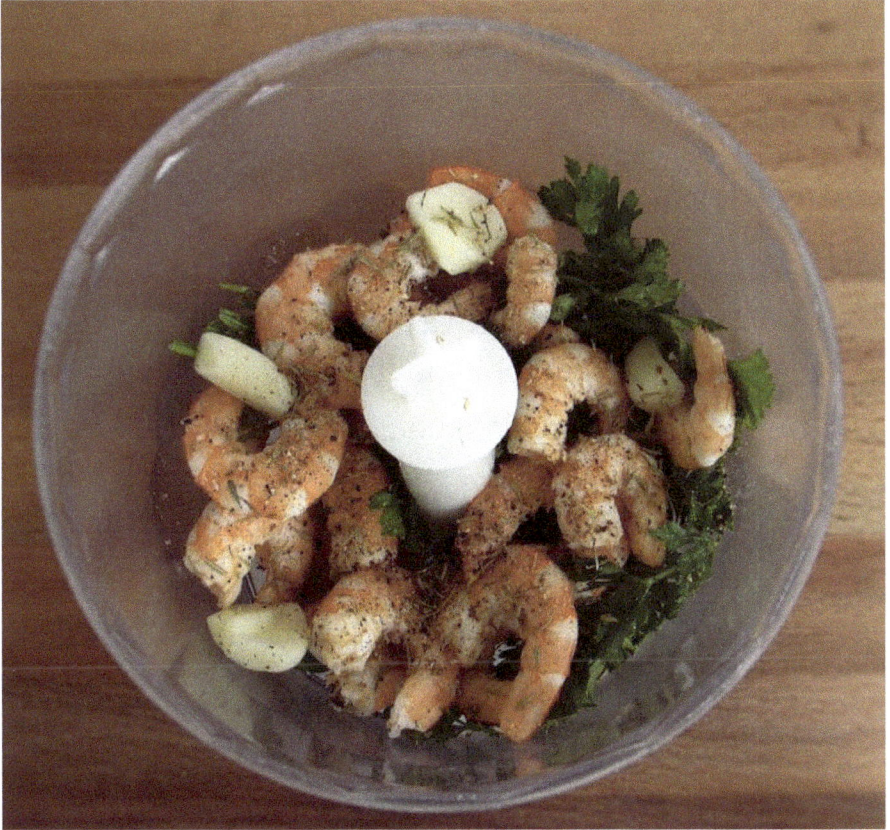

Chili Cumin Cod

Prep time: 10 minutes I **Cooking time:** 14 minutes I
Servings: 4

Ingredients:

- 4 cod fillets, boneless
- ½ pound green beans, trimmed and halved
- 1 tablespoon lime juice
- 1 tablespoon lime zest, grated
- 1 yellow onion, chopped
- 2 tablespoons olive oil
- 1 teaspoon cumin, ground
- 1 teaspoon chili powder
- ½ cup veggie stock
- A pinch of salt and black pepper

Directions:

1. Heat up a pan with the oil over medium-high heat, add the onion, toss and cook for 2 minutes.
2. Add the fish and cook it for 3 minutes on each side.
3. Add the green beans and the rest of the ingredients, toss gently, cook for 7 minutes more, divide between plates and serve.

Nutrition info per serving: calories 220, fat 13, carbs 14.3, fiber 2.3, protein 12

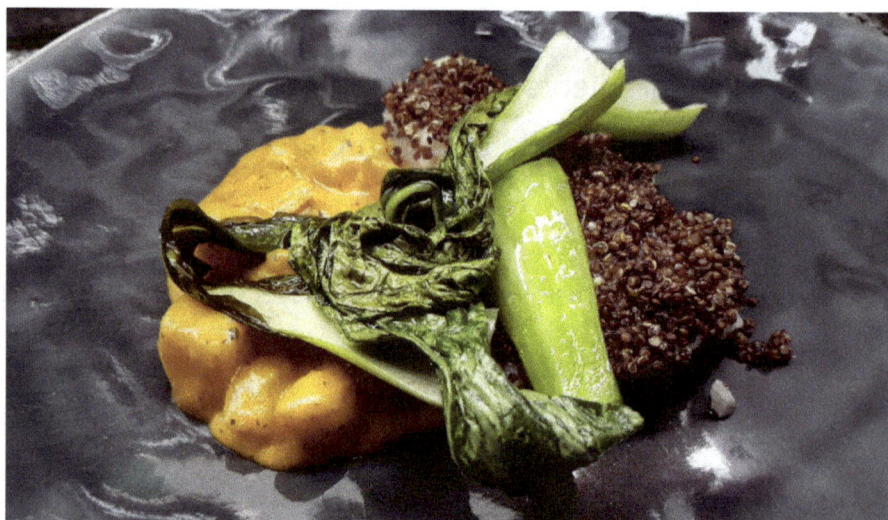

Balsamic Scallops

Prep time: 5 minutes I **Cooking time:** 8 minutes I
Servings: 4

Ingredients:

- 12 scallops
- 1 red onion, sliced
- 2 tablespoons olive oil
- ½ teaspoon garlic, minced
- 2 tablespoons lemon juice
- Black pepper to the taste
- 1 teaspoon balsamic vinegar

Directions:

1. Heat up a pan with the oil over medium heat, add the onion and the garlic and sauté for 2 minutes.
2. Add the scallops and the other ingredients, cook over medium heat for 6 minutes more, divide between plates and serve hot.

Nutrition info per serving: calories 259, fat 8, fiber 3, carbs 5.7, protein 7

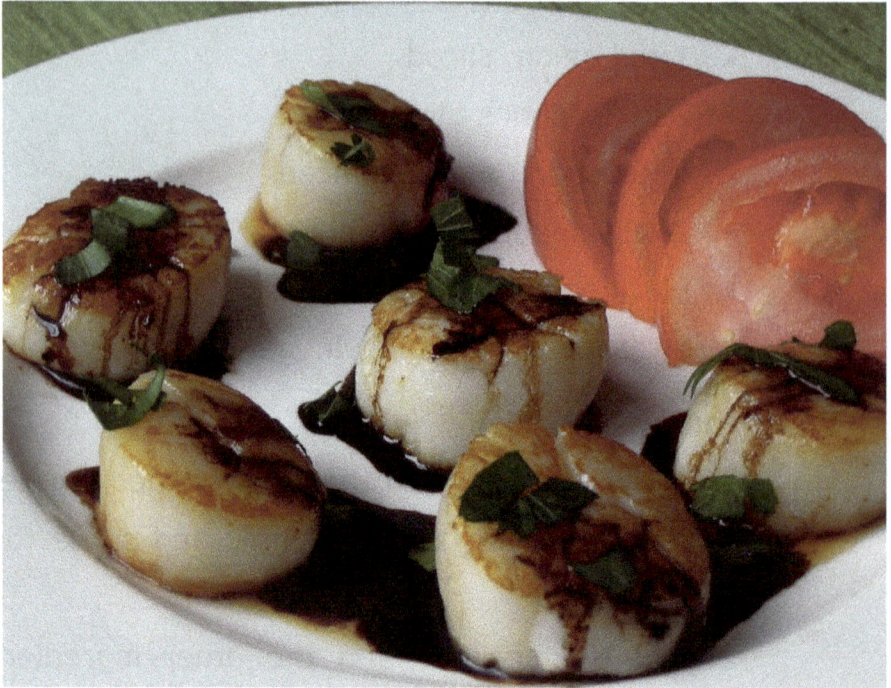

Creamy Lime Sea Bass Mix

Prep time: 10 minutes I **Cooking time:** 14 minutes I
Servings: 4

Ingredients:

- 4 sea bass fillets, boneless
- 1 cup coconut cream
- 1 yellow onion, chopped
- 1 tablespoon lime juice
- 2 tablespoons avocado oil
- 1 tablespoon parsley, chopped
- A pinch of black pepper

Directions:

1. Heat up a pan with the oil over medium heat, add the onion, toss and sauté for 2 minutes.
2. Add the fish and cook it for 4 minutes on each side.
3. Add the rest of the ingredients, cook everything for 4 minutes more, divide between plates and serve.

Nutrition info per serving: calories 283, fat 12.3, fiber 5, carbs 12.5, protein 8

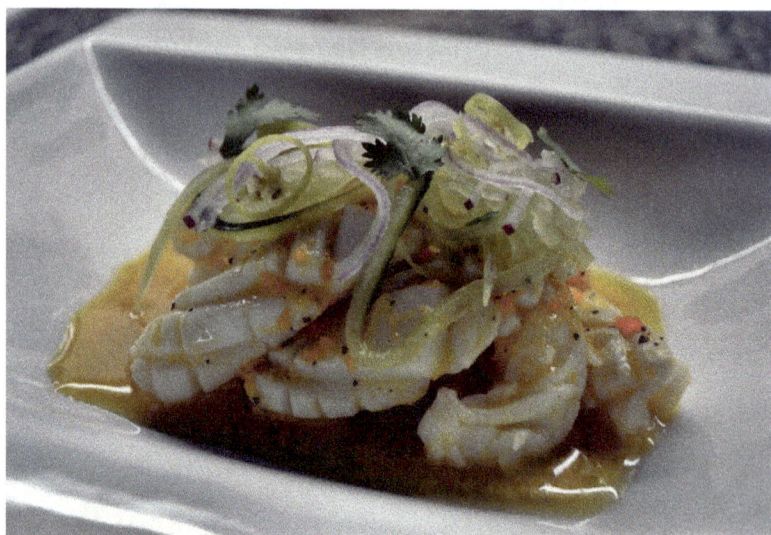

Fish and Mushrooms Mix

Prep time: 10 minutes I **Cooking time:** 13 minutes I
Servings: 4

Ingredients:

- 4 sea bass fillets, boneless
- 2 tablespoons olive oil
- Black pepper to the taste
- ½ cup white mushrooms, sliced
- 1 red onion, chopped
- 2 tablespoons balsamic vinegar
- 3 tablespoons cilantro, chopped

Directions:

1. Heat up a pan with the oil over medium-high heat, add the onion and the mushrooms, stir and cook for 5 minutes.
2. Add the fish and the other ingredients, cook for 4 minutes on each side, divide everything between plates and serve.

Nutrition info per serving: calories 280, fat 12.3, fiber 8, carbs 13.6, protein 14.3

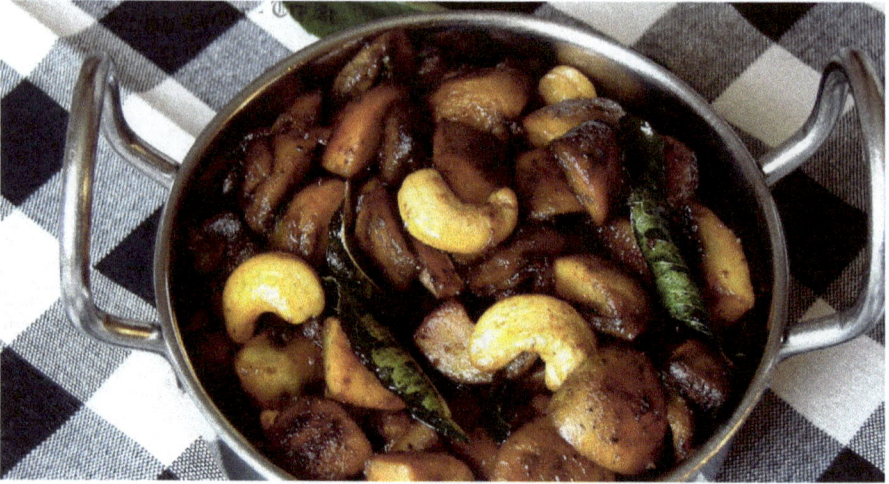

Salmon and Tomato Soup

Prep time: 5 minutes I **Cooking time:** 20 minutes I
Servings: 4

Ingredients:

- 1 pound salmon fillets, boneless, skinless and cubed
- 1 cup yellow onion, chopped
- 2 tablespoons olive oil
- Black pepper to the taste
- 2 cups veggie stock
- 1 and ½ cups tomatoes, chopped
- 1 tablespoon basil, chopped

Directions:

1. Heat up a pot with the oil over medium heat, add the onion, stir and sauté for 5 minutes.
2. Add the salmon and the other ingredients, bring to a simmer and cook over medium heat for 15 minutes.
3. Divide the chowder into bowls and serve.

Nutrition info per serving: calories 250, fat 12.2, fiber 5, carbs 8.5, protein 7

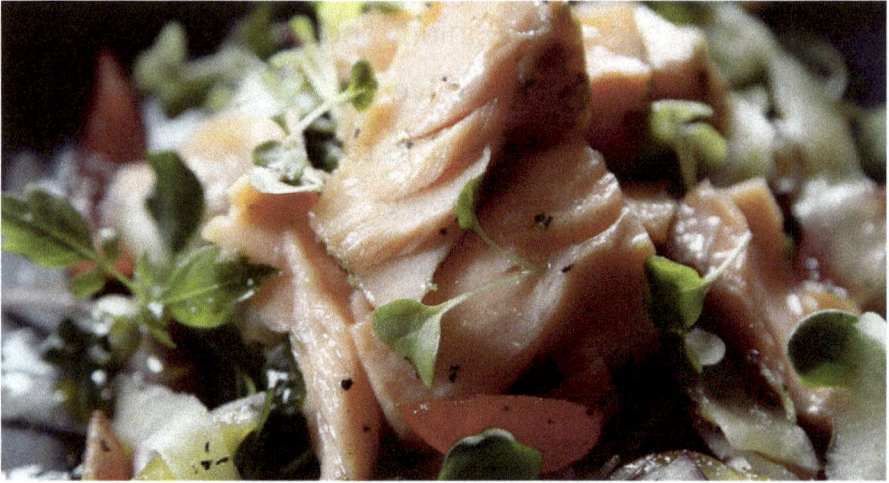

Cinnamon Shrimp

Prep time: 3 minutes I **Cooking time:** 6 minutes I
Servings: 4

Ingredients:

- 1 pound shrimp, peeled and deveined
- 2 tablespoons olive oil
- 1 tablespoon lemon juice
- 1 tablespoon cinnamon, ground
- Black pepper to the taste
- 1 tablespoon cilantro, chopped

Directions:

1. Heat up a pan with the oil over medium heat, add the shrimp, lemon juice and the other ingredients, toss, cook for 6 minutes, divide into bowls and serve.

Nutrition info per serving: calories 205, fat 9.6, fiber 0.4, carbs 2.7, protein 26

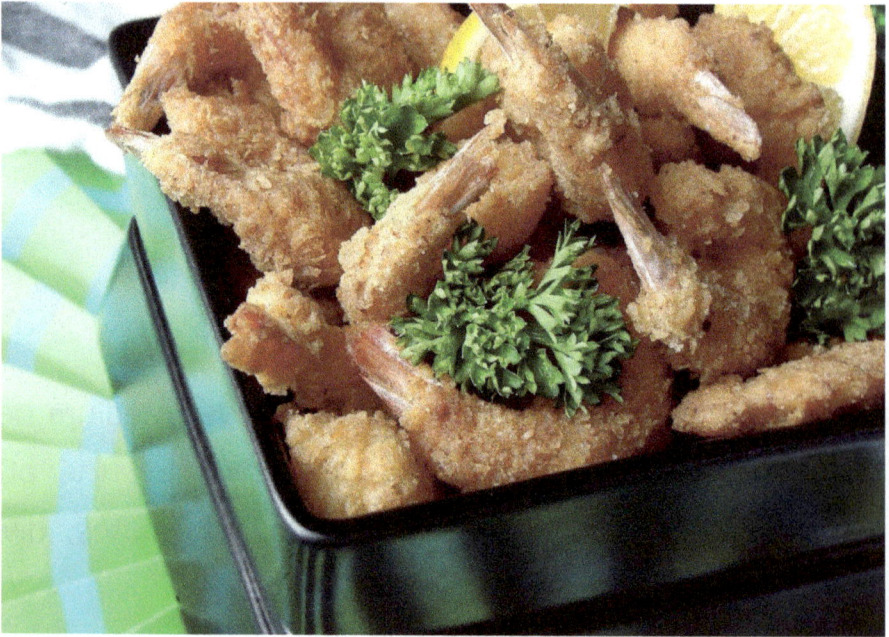

Shrimp and Blueberries Mix

Prep time: 4 minutes I **Cooking time:** 6 minutes I
Servings: 4

Ingredients:

- 1 pound shrimp, peeled and deveined
- ½ cup tomatoes, cubed
- 2 tablespoons olive oil
- 1 tablespoon balsamic vinegar
- ½ cup blueberries, chopped
- Black pepper to the taste

Directions:

1. Heat up a pan with the oil over medium heat, add the shrimp, toss and cook for 3 minutes.
2. Add the rest of the ingredients, toss, cook for 3-4 minutes more, divide into bowls and serve.

Nutrition info per serving: calories 205, fat 9, fiber 0.6, carbs 4, protein 26.2

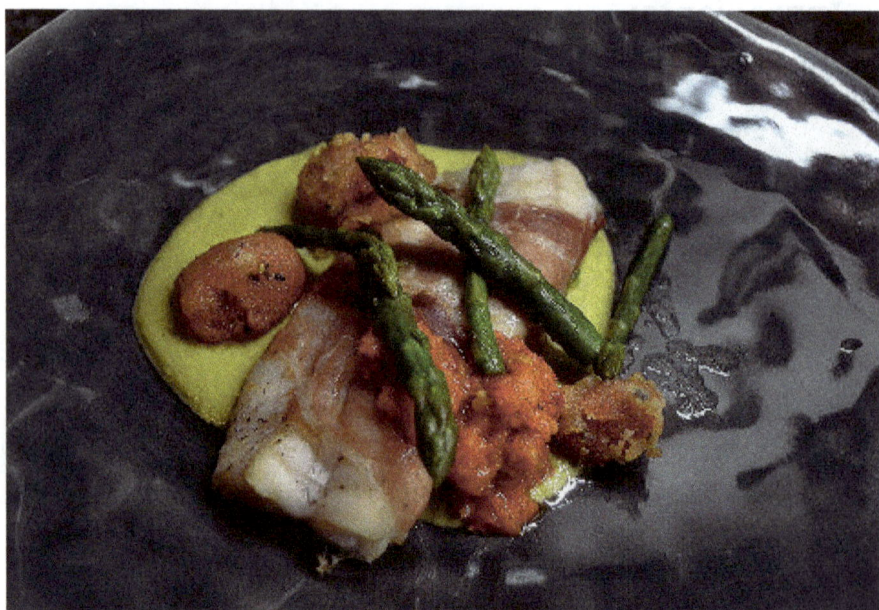

Baked Trout

Prep time: 10 minutes I **Cooking time:** 30 minutes I
Servings: 4

Ingredients:

- 4 trout
- 1 tablespoon lemon zest, grated
- 2 tablespoons olive oil
- 2 tablespoons lemon juice
- A pinch of black pepper
- 2 tablespoons cilantro, chopped

Directions:

1. In a baking dish, combine the fish with the lemon zest and the other ingredients and rub.
2. Bake at 370 degrees F for 30 minutes, divide between plates and serve.

Nutrition info per serving: calories 264, fat 12.3, fiber 5, carbs 7, protein 11

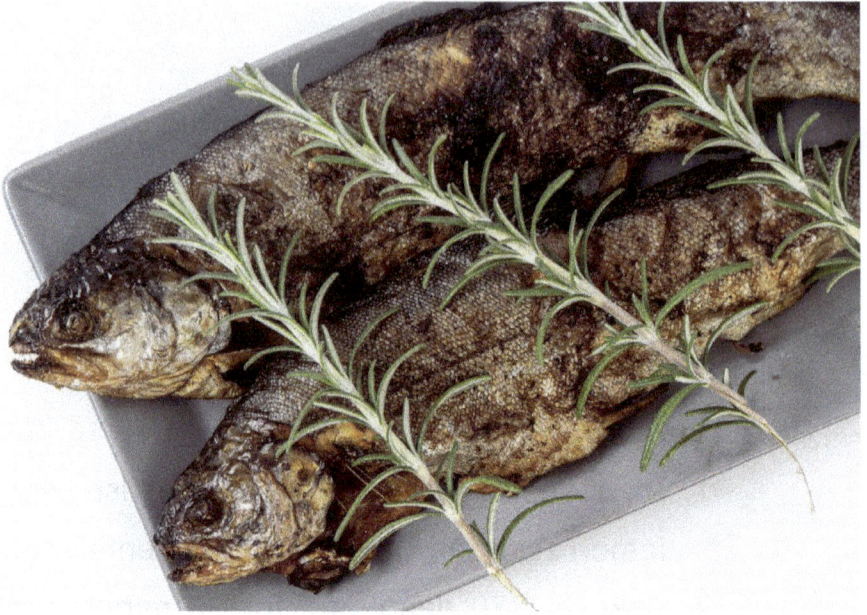

Paprika Scallops

Prep time: 3 minutes I **Cooking time:** 4 minutes I
Servings: 4

Ingredients:

- 12 scallops
- 2 tablespoons olive oil
- Black pepper to the taste
- 2 tablespoons chives, chopped
- 1 tablespoon sweet paprika

Directions:

1. Heat up a pan with the oil over medium heat, add the scallops, paprika and the other ingredients, and cook for 2 minutes on each side.
2. Divide between plates and serve with a side salad.

Nutrition info per serving: calories 215, fat 6, fiber 5, carbs 4.5, protein 11

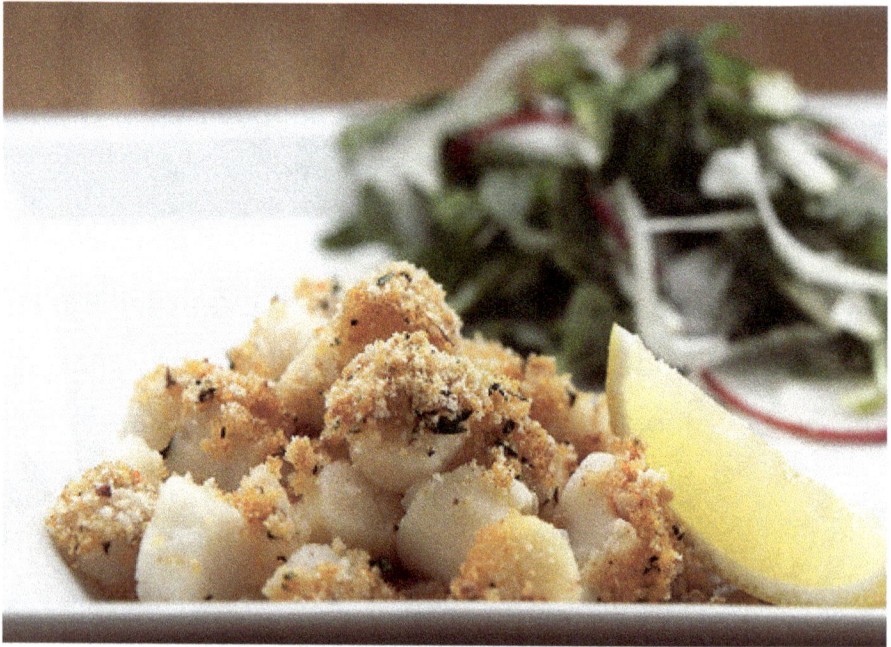

Fish Meatballs

Prep time: 10 minutes I **Cooking time:** 30 minutes I
Servings: 4

Ingredients:

- 2 tablespoons olive oil
- 1 pound tuna, skinless, boneless and minced
- 1 yellow onion, chopped
- ¼ cup chives, chopped
- 1 egg, whisked
- 1 tablespoon coconut flour
- A pinch of salt and black pepper

Directions:

1. In a bowl, mix the tuna with the onion and the other ingredients except the oil, stir well and shape medium meatballs out of this mix.
2. Arrange the meatballs on a baking sheet, grease them with the oil, introduce in the oven at 350 degrees F, cook for 30 minutes, divide between plates and serve.

Nutrition info per serving: calories 291, fat 14.3, fiber 5, carbs 12.4, protein 11

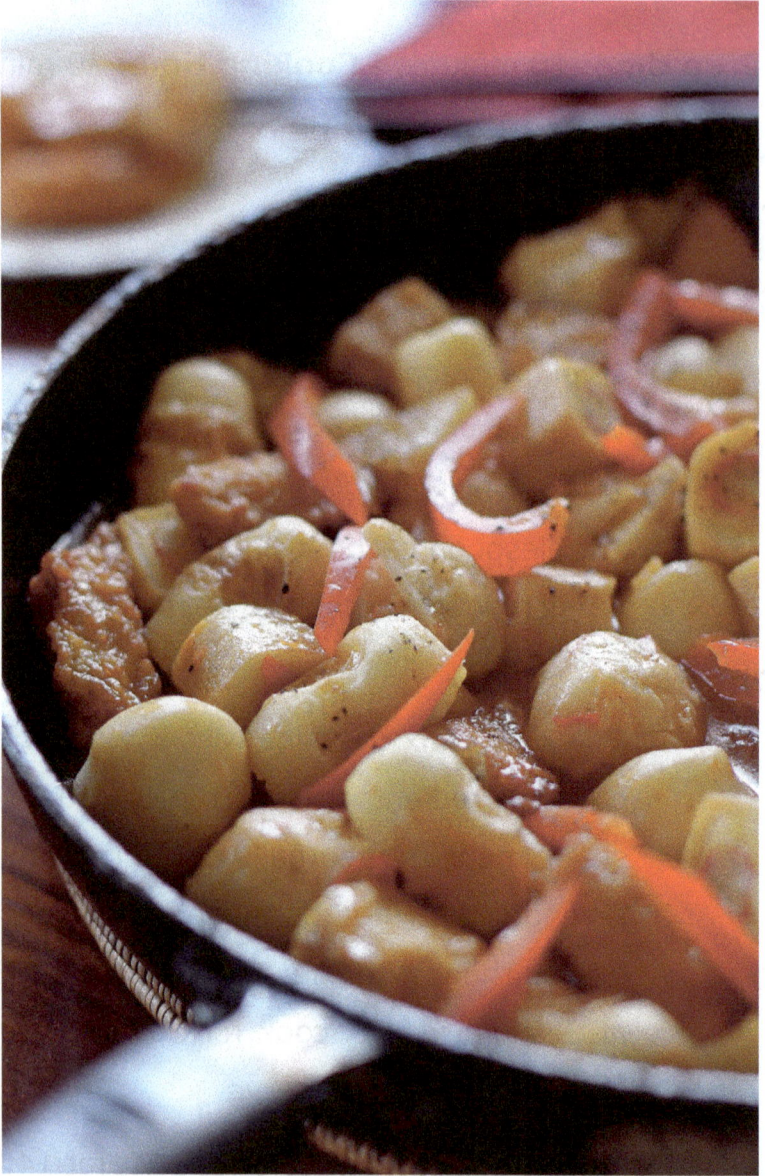

Salmon and Eggplant Pan

Prep time: 10 minutes I **Cooking time:** 12 minutes I
Servings: 4

Ingredients:

- 4 salmon fillets, boneless and roughly cubed
- 2 tablespoons olive oil
- 1 red bell pepper, cut into strips
- 2 eggplants, roughly cubed
- 1 tablespoon lemon juice
- 1 tablespoon dill, chopped
- ¼ cup veggie stock
- 1 teaspoon garlic powder
- A pinch of black pepper

Directions:

1. Heat up a pan with oil over medium-high heat, add the bell pepper and the eggplant, toss and sauté for 3 minutes.
2. Add the salmon and the other ingredients, toss gently, cook everything for 9 minutes more, divide between plates and serve.

Nutrition info per serving: calories 348, fat 18.4, fiber 5.3, carbs 11.9, protein 36.9

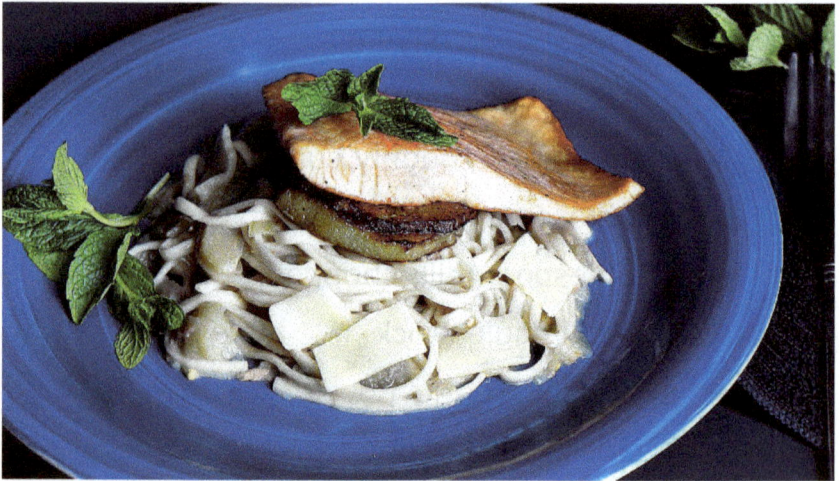

Mustard and Turmeric Cod

Prep time: 10 minutes I **Cooking time:** 25 minutes I
Servings: 4

Ingredients:

- 4 cod fillets, skinless and boneless
- A pinch of black pepper
- 1 teaspoon ginger, grated
- 1 tablespoon mustard
- 2 tablespoons olive oil
- 1 teaspoon thyme, dried
- ¼ teaspoon cumin, ground
- 1 teaspoon turmeric powder
- ¼ cup cilantro, chopped
- 1 cup veggie stock
- 3 garlic cloves, minced

Directions:

1. In a roasting pan, combine the cod with the black pepper, ginger and the other ingredients, toss gently and bake at 380 degrees F for 25 minutes.
2. Divide the mix between plates and serve.

Nutrition info per serving: calories 176, fat 9, fiber 1, carbs 3.7, protein 21.2

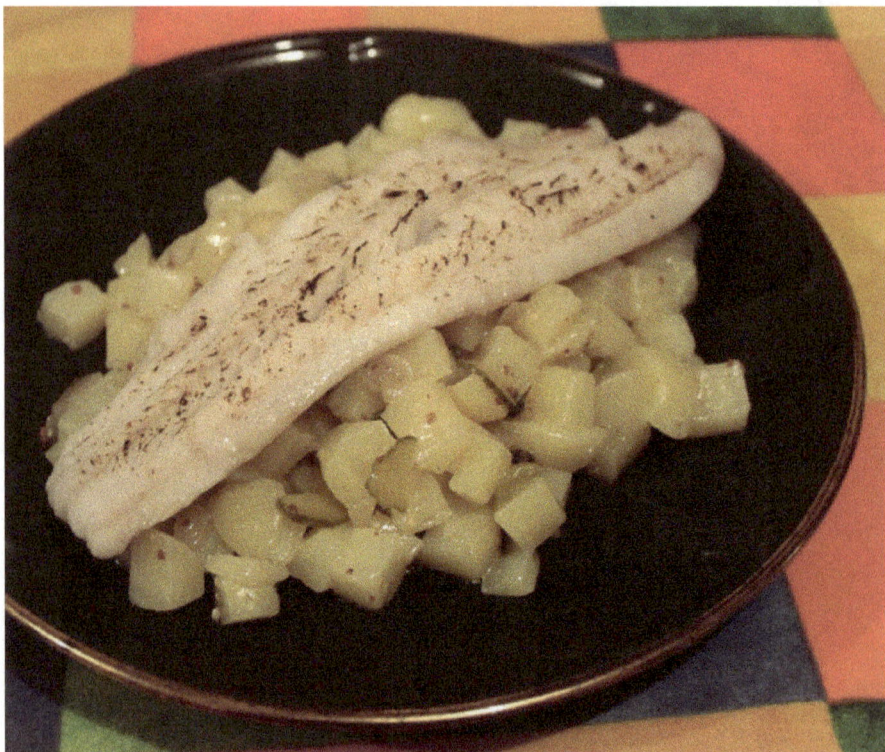

Shrimp and Walnuts

Prep time: 10 minutes I **Cooking time:** 14 minutes I
Servings: 4

Ingredients:

- 1/2 cup walnuts, chopped
- 1 pound shrimp, peeled and deveined
- Black pepper to the taste
- 2 tablespoons olive oil
- 1 red onion, chopped
- 2 garlic cloves, minced
- 1 cup coconut cream

Directions:

1. Heat up a pan with the oil over medium heat, add the onion, garlic and the walnuts, toss and cook for 4 minutes.
2. Add the shrimp and the other ingredients, toss, simmer over medium heat for 10 minutes, divide everything into bowls and serve.

Nutrition info per serving: calories 225, fat 6, fiber 3.4, carbs 8.6, protein 8

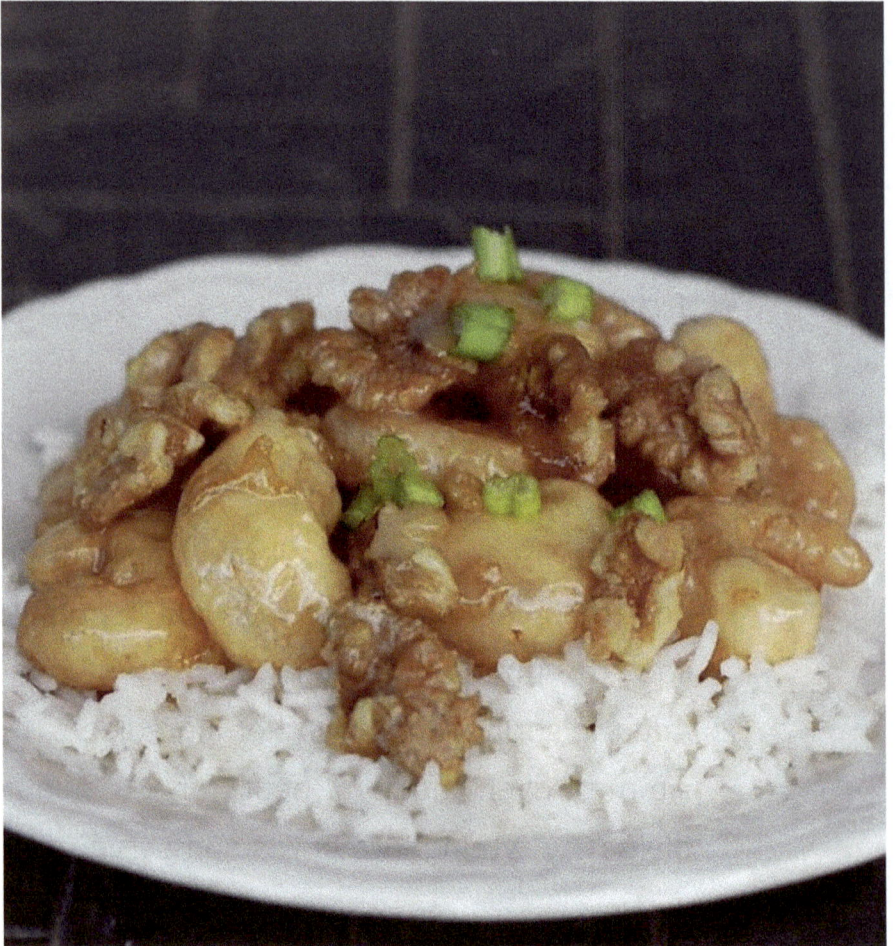

Cod and Corn

Prep time: 10 minutes I **Cooking time:** 20 minutes I
Servings: 4

Ingredients:

- 1 yellow onion, chopped
- 2 tablespoons olive oil
- ½ cup chicken stock
- 4 cod fillets, boneless, skinless
- Black pepper to the taste
- 1 cup corn

Directions:

1. Heat up a pot with the oil over medium heat, add the onion, stir and sauté fro 4 minutes.
2. Add the fish and cook it for 3 minutes on each side.
3. Add the corn and the other ingredients, cook everything for 10 minutes more, divide between plates and serve.

Nutrition info per serving: calories 240, fat 8.4, fiber 2.7, carbs 7.6, protein 14

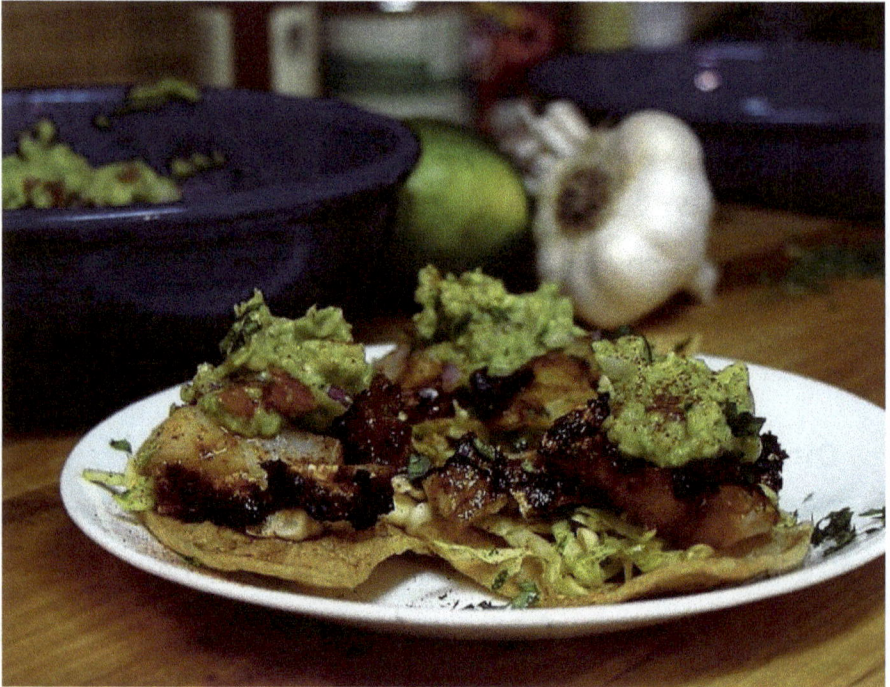

Shrimp and Mussels Mix

Prep time: 5 minutes I **Cooking time:** 12 minutes I
Servings: 4

Ingredients:

- 1 pound mussels, scrubbed
- ½ cup chicken stock
- 1 pound shrimp, peeled and deveined
- 2 shallots, minced
- 1 cup cherry tomatoes, cubed
- 2 garlic cloves, minced
- 1 tablespoon olive oil
- Juice of 1 lemon

Directions:

1. Heat up a pan with the oil over medium heat, add the shallots and the garlic and sauté for 2 minutes.
2. Add the shrimp, mussels and the other ingredients, cook everything over medium heat for 10 minutes, divide into bowls and serve.

Nutrition info per serving: calories 240, fat 4.9, fiber 2.4, carbs 11.6, protein 8

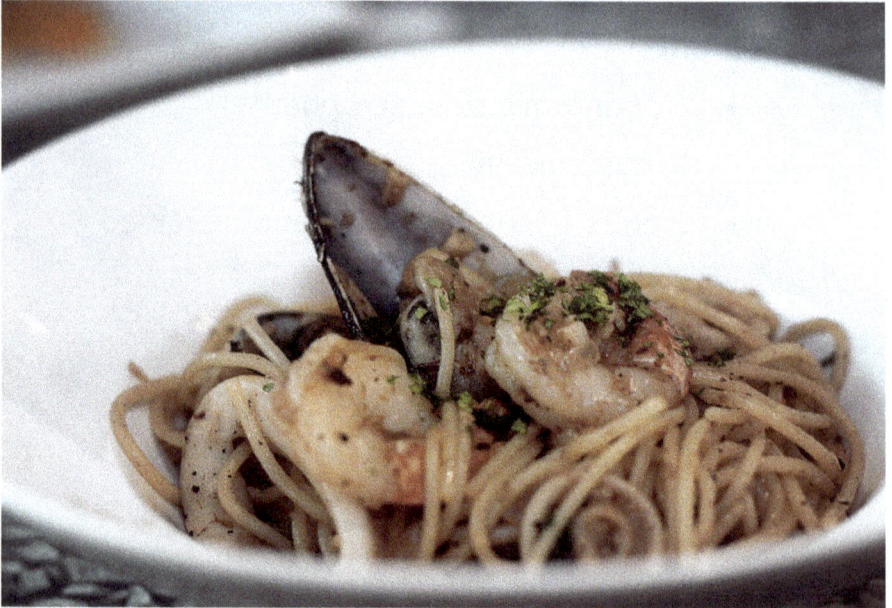

www.ingramcontent.com/pod-product-compliance
Lightning Source LLC
Chambersburg PA
CBHW050753030426
42336CB00012B/1802